Mastering Patient Flow
More Ideas to Increase Efficiency and Earnings
2nd Edition

By Elizabeth Woodcock, MBA, FACMPE

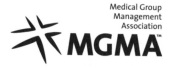

Medical Group
Management
Association

Medical Group Management Association
104 Inverness Terrace East
Englewood, CO   80112
877.275.6462
Web site: www.mgma.com

Medical Group Management (MGMA) publications are intended to provide current and accurate information and are designed to assist readers in becoming more familiar with the subject matter covered. Such publications are distributed with the understanding that MGMA does not render any legal, accounting or other professional advice that may be construed as specifically applicable to individual situations. No representations or warranties are made concerning the application of legal or other principles discussed by the authors to any specific factual situation, nor is any prediction made concerning how any particular judge, government official, or other person will interpret or apply such principles. Specific factual situations should be discussed with professional advisors.

Cover photo courtesy of CopyDisk

Item # 6072

ISBN: 1-56829-228-7

Printed in the United States of America
10 9 8 7 6 5 4 3 2 1

Contents

Chapter 4. Scheduling   87

Chapter 5. Registration   147

Chapter 6. Waiting   179

Chapter 7. The Patient Encounter   195

Chapter 8. Checkout   223

About the author

Elizabeth W. Woodcock, MBA, FACMPE, has visited countless medical practices in search of how to master patient flow. Believing that efficiency and earnings can be achieved, she presents practical advice sure to create the environment in which every medical practice can improve the patient flow process.

Educated at Duke University (BA) and the Wharton School of Business (MBA), Elizabeth has traveled the country as an industry researcher, operations consultant and expert presenter. Currently Director of Knowledge Management for Physicians Practice, Inc., Elizabeth has focused on medical practice operations throughout her career. She has served as a consultant with the Medical Group Management Association Health Care Consulting Group, group practice services administrator at the University of Virginia Health Services Foundation and a senior associate at the Health Care Advisory Board.

Elizabeth is a Fellow in the American College of Medical Practice Executives® (ACMPE®) and is a member of the ACMPE Board of Directors. In addition to co-authoring *Operating Policies and Procedures Manual for Medical Groups* (1st and 2nd Editions), Elizabeth is a frequent contributor to national health care publications. She currently resides in Atlanta, Georgia, with her husband and two children.

About the editor

Robert Redling, MS, is senior writer at the Medical Group Management Association. A graduate of San Diego State University and the University of Kansas, Lawrence, where he earned his master's of science in journalism, Robert has been a speechwriter for the American Academy of Family Physicians, a legislative correspondent for United Press International, and a reporter for the Wyoming Daily Eagle, Cheyenne. He currently lives in Kansas City, Missouri.

Preface

On the surface, mastering patient flow may seem easy. But our everyday tasks — scheduling, answering the telephones and so on — are filled with variability. It is important to remember that the "flow" we manage is people's lives.

It is with this notion that I write the second edition of this book. I have learned that the key to mastering patient flow is to have many tools in your resource toolbox. The more tools you have, the greater your flexibility in responding to the new challenges that each day brings. For example, we do not serve our patients well by sticking to inflexible scheduling approaches designed more for the convenience of clinicians and staff, instead of the patient's convenience.

Mastering Patient Flow: Second Edition is your resource toolbox for medical practice operations. Not every idea will work for you, nor will every suggestion work every day. The key is to have many ideas — tools, in other words — to use when and where you need them. We must master many tools to survive and thrive.

MGMA is pleased to be a partner in opening this resource toolbox for medical groups.

Acknowledgments

Since the publishing of the first edition of this book, I have brought two beautiful babies into this world. It is to them – Joseph Cade and Estelle McLaughlin – that I dedicate this book. My hope for you is to be as blessed with the support of friends and colleagues as I have.

Elizabeth W. Woodcock, MBA, FACMPE

Chapter 1

INTRODUCTION

Who should read this book?

This book is a manual to help medical practices manage their patient flow to improve efficiency and earnings. The ideas, descriptions and resources in this updated, second edition will be of value whether you are new to practice management, are changing duties, or face new challenges.

If you are relatively new to practice management, use this book to quickly get up to speed on the fundamentals of managing the operations of a medical practice. If you are more experienced, use this book as a quick reference and refresher course to revisit many familiar concepts from a new perspective.

This book is neither meant to be exclusively for a large practice nor for a small practice; neither specialists nor primary care. It is an all-purpose primer on improving patient flow to increase efficiency and earnings in a medical practice. Readers at all levels of experience and in all types and sizes of medical practices will find handy tools to monitor current operations and discover areas to improve. Even if you've read the first edition, you'll find many new ideas in this revised and updated edition.

Whether you are a nurse, physician or administrator, this book is valuable to you.

Why should you read this book?

Maybe you picked up this book because you want to improve your practice's revenue. Maybe you want to improve patient satisfaction. Maybe you want to boost staff and physician performance, morale and productivity. So, what's standing in your way? Often, it is the bottlenecks in patient flow. As you strive to increase your business and serve your patients better, don't find yourself struggling to retain their business because of a disgruntled receptionist, a telephone system that always rings busy, or lengthy wait times.

In this book, we will walk through every aspect of your practice as it impacts the patient. By evaluating a medical practice quantitatively and qualitatively, we can discover and remove logjams that disrupt the flow of patients through the practice. Smoother patient flow will help your practice generate more cash at lower cost (i.e., lower overhead), achieve better patient satisfaction, retain physicians and employees, and become more competitive in its market and more resilient over the long term. In other words, better patient flow will empower your practice to become stronger.

Loyalty used to keep patients coming back to your physicians, but today's patients are far less tolerant of an inefficient office, no matter how good the quality of care you provide. The same goes for payers and referring physicians when they repeatedly hear patients complain about your practice. Patients, referring physicians, payers and your other customers relate your quality of service to your quality of care. If your service is sub-optimal, you will lose those patients. Let's make sure that you don't by mastering the patient flow process!

Why this book is different

Many practice management books are structured around the various aspects of running a practice from the point of view of the manager or the physician. This book attacks many of the same issues but from the perspective of that most important person in your medical practice: the patient. The book's chapters parallel the contact points between patients and your practice with the end result – I hope – being a new perspective on how patients flow through the practice and, where the logjams are that may impede that "flow" and cost you money.

This book differs from many others because it acknowledges that there is no one right way for a medical practice to function. Yet, there are steps that all practices can take to improve efficiency and patient flow while providing exceptional customer service. This, indeed, is the ideal patient encounter.

Rather than tackle every activity of a medical practice, this book focuses on the functions surrounding (and, too often, slowing down) the flow of patients – from telephones to scheduling to provision of care to checkout. To supplement the patient flow process, I have included sections on the physician's time and costs, both of which are critical to creating an efficient and cost-effective patient flow process. New to this second edition is a section on technology – a business function closely tied to the efficiency and effectiveness of medical practice operations.

The issue of receivables management is addressed as it relates to the patient flow process, to include patient registration and charge entry (at checkout). Due to the complexity of the issues, there is not a comprehensive coverage of billing and collections, nor the related subject of compliance. Although these subjects are not addressed in-depth, make no mistake, they are critical. Why? Because each member of your staff, including your physicians, is a member of "the billing office" and the "compliance team." Thus, when appropriate, I have incorporated tips on the billing process, particularly as it relates to registration, charge capture and charge entry.

How to use this book

Since this book is organized around the natural flow of patients through your practice, I hope you will follow this path from beginning to end. However, if you wish to focus on only one function, then jump ahead to that section.

Each section is organized around a function in the operations process. After introducing you to the most important asset in your practice – your physician's time, we will explore ways to create the ideal patient encounter to improve efficiency and earnings in your practice. I say "we" because you will get the greatest use from this book by substituting your practice's data where possible in the examples and worksheets.

The chapters are outlined as follows:

Chapter 2. The Physician's Time: We begin with a look at your practice's most valuable asset – the *time* of your physician or any other billable provider. This provides a meaningful introduction to the patient flow process and the recognition of the necessity of maximizing this asset.

Chapter 3. Telephones: We couldn't discuss patient flow without highlighting telephones, as this is your patients' first impression of your office operations. This process is explored through managing patients' demand, as well as a comprehensive overview of telephone systems and features, and telephony applications.

Chapter 4. Scheduling: The patient flow process is created from scheduling. Following a brief overview of scheduling, we take an in-depth look at advanced access scheduling and controlling no-shows.

Chapter 5. Registration: The patients' presentation to the practice will be explored in this chapter, with an in-depth look at pre-visit processes.

Chapter 6. Waiting: Always a part of the flow process in a medical practice, we take a good look at waiting, improving it and ways to manage it.

Chapter 7. The Patient Encounter: The patient flow process revolves around the actual provision of care – the patient encounter. In this chapter, physician efficiency is explored in depth as we follow patients from the reception area into the clinical area until they move to checkout.

Chapter 8. Checkout: The checkout process varies among specialties but the core objectives remain the same. We explore these processes from charge entry to referrals.

Chapter 9. Technology: New technology can help the patient flow process, but it also can hurt it. The chapter walks you through vital new technologies that can improve patient flow and shows you how to evaluate them.

Chapter 10. Fundamental Financials: Practice operations cannot be managed without an understanding of the core financial concepts embedded in the operations of a medical practice. A concise but informative look at the numbers will establish a solid base from which to leap from ideas gathered in this book to implementing operations changes in your practice.

Chapter 11. Summing Up: We conclude with a summary of the most important concepts discussed in our journey through the perfect patient encounter.

Self-assessment tools and worksheets are provided. Also integrated into each chapter are case studies and advice from your peers.

To make it easier for you to revisit this book later on and quickly find what you need, more detailed information about the processes of patient flow appears in separate boxes.

These boxes are:

"Getting started"
Specific questions to ask or materials/resources to assemble before changing key office functions.

"Steps to get you there"
Actions you need to take in changing a key office function.

"Things to consider"
Issues or logistics to consider as you attempt to make changes.

"Case studies"
How another practice solved a key process problem and improved patient flow in the practice.

"You know..."
Hints that something is or is not working in your practice.

"Words of wisdom"
Just that. Handy tips and insights from the author, industry experts, health care leaders and practice managers.

"Key concepts"
Explanations that give perspective on key concepts mentioned in the text.

Advanced concepts appear at the end of each section for experienced readers – and those who are willing to innovate – to learn more about the process being discussed.

After you read this book

Before you embark on operational changes, look at your practice and consider the variables that can affect your ability to change critical processes affecting patient flow:

Your Facility:

The physical layout of your facility has a huge impact on operations. Can you afford to modify your floorplan? If your nurses' station is distant from your front office, transferring a patient's record from the front to the clinical area and announcing the patient's arrival to the clinical team become more complicated. You may have to use an elaborate lighting system, convex mirrors, or simply walk down the hall. Indeed, the physical attributes of your facility will dictate your operations to an extent.

Your Practice Management System:

Whether it is manual, automated or somewhere in between, the system you use to manage information in your practice dictates some operational processes. If you schedule from a book, then handling appointments from callers and scheduling follow-up appointments with patients checking out should both reside in the same physical location. If you are computerized, can your system post and suspend copayments without first posting a charge? If not, then collecting payments prior to the time of service will be complicated.

Your "That's The Way We've Always Done It" Factor:

This is the most common and most dangerous of all variables. As you make changes in your practice, be on the look out for those words. When you hear them, look upon it as an opportunity. This is the one variable which requires no walls to be constructed or software modules to be purchased, only that attitudes change. The assessment tools in this book will give you some of the ammunition you need to overcome this most difficult variable.

This book will be a useful resource but, rest assured, some of your attempted changes will fail. In fact, if you don't experience some failures, then you might not be trying hard enough to make change.

The path to success is paved with opportunities and challenges: failing at some initiatives is a natural process and should not be looked down upon. There is no right way to operate a practice. Creating the ideal patient flow in your practice is difficult, but we believe that it should be your goal.

There are so many ideas in this book that it may seem overwhelming. For best results, create an action plan to master patient flow in your office. Divide your practice into teams each representing a chapter in this book. Issue a challenge for each team to make at least three improvements, and offer a small prize to the team with the ideas that make the most significant impact.

Even if you only pick up a few ideas to help your practice improve the patient flow process, then this book will have done its job!

THE PHYSICIAN'S TIME

Key Chapter Lessons

> Recognize your physician's time as the practice's greatest asset

> Understand the applicability of leverage to your practice

> Categorize your physician's time

> Discover how office design and technology can save time

> Learn to maximize productive time by reducing wasted and delegated time

> Analyze the contribution of productivity improvement to earnings

> Understand the value of appropriate staffing

> Use strategies to help new physicians perform better

Advanced Concepts

> Average Value of a Customer (AVC)

> New physicians

> Going solo

Your most valuable asset

Before we leap into examining the patient's experience with your practice, let's explore a fundamental concept behind your operations. Take this little test to see if you understand the value of your practice's most important asset.

Who can bill for a service in your practice?

a. telephone operator

b. medical assistant

c. physician

d. biller

e. office manager

Of course the answer is "c," the physician. The vast majority of the revenue produced by your practice is a function of the physician's time[1].

In a fee-for-service environment, if a physician doesn't bill for a service, he or she doesn't get paid for that service. In a capitated environment, inefficient use of a physician's time can translate into a smaller patient panel that, in turn, reduces the group's PMPM (per-member, per-month) payments. The name of the game is to leverage your physicians' time so that they are as productive as possible in contributing to your patients' care – and your bottom line.

Physicians are the medical practice's key to volume. But they also are the practice's most costly resource and the resource most difficult to assess in terms of revenue versus cost. The critical question is, can the physician bring in more money to the practice than it must spend on the fixed costs of supporting the physician's activities?

---

1. Not all practices rely on physicians as the sole billable providers. Many function with midlevel providers such as nurse practitioners, physician assistants, nurse anesthetists and other clinicians. Instead of listing each profession when discussing the role of a billable provider, this book will refer to a "physician." It is important to note that if your practice employs billable providers other than physicians, their professional titles can be substituted for "physician" throughout the book.

How can you learn to control and, even, predict costs when they are never fixed and produce variable amounts of revenue? If you think of your physicians in terms of their time, then you can easily see that this is the single most expensive resource in your practice. That's why, as we go through the steps of improving patient flow, I will try to view the usefulness of the improvements in terms of whether or not they maximize the physicians' time.

Physician productivity

Physicians' time can be divided into three categories: productive, wasted and delegated. The key to success is to maximize the productive time, eliminate the wasted time and hire support staff to handle what can be delegated.

The physician's minutes add up

At first, redesigning the patient flow process may seem like a lot of work for little return. What's the use of freeing up just a minute or two of the physician's time per patient visit? Multiply those salvaged minutes or fractions of a minute by the number of patients your physicians see each day, week, or month. You can see that saving a minute here and there can add up to hours over the year. Hours in which the physician could be seeing additional patients and producing revenue for the practice without the stress of working longer days.

Since the primary financial driver of profits in a medical practice is how the physician's time is used, that resource – the physician's time – is where to focus many of your efforts to smooth patient flow. Don't make the mistake of devoting hundreds of hours of staff time and, perhaps, hundreds or thousands of dollars on top of that, to improve a process that doesn't help the physicians become more productive in terms of time. Think in terms of what can help the physician and patient work better together.

Examine the physician's non-clinical tasks

The best way to quickly maximize the amount of time the physician can spend with a patient is to look for ways to reduce the amount of time the physician has to spend on non-clinical administrative tasks before, during and after a patient visit.

Do you see your physician spending time to track down charts, filling out long forms instead of using templates to order diagnostic tests, or going through a medical staff directory to find a referring physician's telephone number?

Is there a relatively modest change that can be made in your facility's floor plan or can a nurses' station or computer terminal be moved or redesigned so it will save the physician a few extra steps? The cost to make such changes can be recouped several times over if doing so makes more efficient use of the time of a physician or any billable provider.

Check with vendors to see if there's a way to shorten or simplify the way physicians interact with the practice management system or electronic medical record. Easy-to-access electronic templates for progress notes, prescriptions, referrals or other forms can encourage your physicians to use electronic instead of handwritten forms. If that saves time for the physician, then it's a good option to explore.

If possible, spend a half a day observing your physicians as they interact with other staff before and after patient visits. Take notes of what tasks they perform, how long each task takes, and how long it takes for them to walk to or prepare for the next task. Note times by the minute. You might quickly see a way to improve a simple process that is eating up your physician's time, such as waiting to transfer paperwork from the back to the front office or chaperoning patients from one area to another.

Key concepts

Capitation: A methodology of payment for physician services that is based on a flat fee to manage the care of a patient. In contrast to fee-for-service, what you are paid a fee for each service, capitation transfers the risk of care management to the physician. That is, if the patient covered under capitation never sees or communicates with the practice during the year, the payment is all profit. However, the next patient could require a monthly visit to monitor his or her condition, plus supporting telephone time.

Contribution margin: The revenue generated by an additional volume of services minus the variable costs to produce the volume equals the "contribution margin." For example, an in-house lab generates $20,000 in revenue and incurs $5,000 in variable expenses to perform an additional number of tests. Thus, the lab has produced a contribution margin of $15,000 to help cover fixed expenses. In general, when the contribution margin is positive, performing additional services is a good financial decision.

Leverage: The ability to use a resource to increase the value of an asset. For example, leveraging a physician's time by having a nurse return a portion of the calls allows the physician to spend more time with that day's patients. While the nurse answers the telephone calls, the physician can generate more revenue by seeing the next patient. *(This definition simplifies the twin issues of operating and financial leverage. Operating leverage refers to the extent a business commits itself to higher levels of fixed costs. Financial leverage refers to the extent to which a business gets its cash resources from debt as opposed to equity.)*

Panel: The number of active patients that a physician manages. Typically defined as the number of patients seen in the past 36 months, panel sizes run as low as 500 to a high of 6,000, depending upon the physician and the specialty. Panel size is sometimes used to describe the workload of the practice because having more active patients in the panel means more visits, more telephone calls, more refill requests, etc.

Per-member, per-month (PMPM): The amount of payment made in capitated relationships (see "capitation") for physician services. Insurance companies make a monthly payment ($.50 to $20) on behalf of each of their covered beneficiaries for physicians to manage the care of that patient.

Relative value units (RVUs): The work unit of the Resource-based Relative Value Scale (RBRVS), which is the methodology chosen by the Centers for Medicare and Medicaid Services (CMS) to pay physicians for Medicare services. There is an RVU associated with each current procedural terminology (CPT) code, and the scale of all of the codes is published each fall. RVUs are used by many practices as a measurement of productivity because the scale is based on the work, practice expense and malpractice associated with each code. Moreover, the scale is identical across the country, making benchmarking easy.

Space is important factor in productivity

Research proves that the bigger a medical practice gets, the more operationally inefficient it becomes. Why? Because physicians and staff must walk more steps in a larger practice. It sounds trite, but it's true.

The offices of a solo physician who has barely 1,000 square feet of office space may feel cramped, but she can get from the front office to an exam room and back again in mere seconds.

On the opposite end of the scale are the physicians who build an expansive suite of offices that feature long, wide hallways, spacious exam rooms and physician offices located on a separate floor. In these practices, a walk from the front office to farthest exam room seems to take 10 minutes. While that facility may look pretty, those extra footsteps gobble many additional minutes a day. And the cost of those extra minutes will add up to real money very quickly, especially if physicians are the ones who have to make these hikes.

In most practices, physicians spend way too much time walking around. Consider this: Is there a CPT code for walking an encounter form to the front desk? What about accompanying a patient to checkout, or escorting patients to the bathroom? Of course not.

The most efficient physicians consider their suite of exam rooms – usually, three – to be their "playing field." Unless there is an emergency, they remain on the field. This not only saves steps – and time – but it keeps them focused. Put a piece of tape on the ground around your physician's "field." Spend a day shadowing the physician to measure how much time they spend on the field and off. You'll be amazed that the answer is often more time is spent off the field than on it. Change this, and you'll improve your efficiency – guaranteed.

Extra steps reduce physician efficiency

Suppose your practice is one of those where the physicians walk each patient's encounter form to the front desk out of fear that the patient will wander off with the form and never be seen again.

Now, suppose it takes each physician 60 seconds to complete the walk to and from the front office. A physician who saw 30 patients a day would spend an additional 30 minutes a day just carrying forms back and forth. Of course, the physician would start batching some of the errands whether you wanted him to or not, but that would still add up to enough time at the end of the day for him to see one more patient, or at least catch up on other tasks and go home on time and little less stressed.

If this practice had 10 physicians, then the revenue lost due to those extra steps would cost the practice significant income by the end of the year.

Co-location and pods

What can you do to make your office space more efficient for the physicians as well as the staff? For starters, review the processes that make physicians take too many unnecessary steps between work areas. Then, try "co-location," which is bringing the right people and resources together strategically to perform their jobs faster and more efficiently. Use rearrangement of workspace, better adaptation of technology or both to achieve optimal co-location.

The 1990s was the decade of centralization and compartmentalization. Everything from billing offices to telephone operations was combined and given its own physical space. Although this achieved some economies of scale, efficiency was compromised because employees were separated from each other and, often, from the resources they needed to do their jobs and the communication that was essential to getting the job done.

A good alternative to the compartmentalization trend is physical co-location. Group staff and physicians together in workstations where they can perform all administrative functions from scheduling to billing. This type of grouping tends to occur naturally in very small medical practices.

These "pods" work well because communication between the team members is direct and everyone has a pulse on how the day is going. Messaging delays are decreased because the person who takes a message can quickly find the answer or locate someone does. Scheduling is optimized because the scheduler understands the ebb and flow of the day. Clinical staff know the patients and can more easily assist them. Some medical groups have gone so far as to place medical records in the pods to give staff more immediate access to patients' information.

But what if you can't rearrange the workspace to build the ideal work unit? Turn to technology. An electronic medical record makes the transition to pods even easier by eliminating the question of distributing paper charts to each pod. Even minor technology can make a big difference. For example, if you see nurses walking back and forth to the fax machine to pick up refill requests, put a fax machine at the nurses' station.

Many medical groups use e-mail, cell phones, pagers, personal digital assistants, two-way radios, walkie-talkies, colored lights and other electronic tools to help staff communicate to each other within the practice. Some practice management systems have options that can improve internal communication such as arrival notification or patient flow modules.

Today's technologies allow information to be transmitted on a real-time basis. Technology-based co-location can be more efficient than physical co-location if it empowers staff to communicate with each other without taking any steps.

Why pay your staff and your physicians to walk the hallways? Saving them steps pays off in better use of the physician's time, which, as we explore elsewhere in this chapter, isn't cheap.

...you're wasting physicians' time when...

...you see them walking *around* looking for something or somebody to help. If your workflow forces physicians to walk forms, messages or even patients up and down long hallways then you are losing money. Take a day to watch how many steps they take. As you do, keep the following points in mind:

- Do physicians walk patients to the exit as they leave? It's always a nice touch but no patient is going to discuss serious medical issues in the hallway and it certainly isn't in the best interest of preserving the patient's privacy. Even if they are willing, since these conversations are usually not documented, they cannot be considered when coding for the visit. Thus, you can't bill for this "escorting."

Instead, guide physicians into giving patients a kind goodbye as they leave the exam room. If patients tend to get lost in your facility trying to find their way out, consider a redesign, place more signs in the hallways or ask a staff member to escort them.

- Do physicians often leave the exam room to look for missing forms or supplies? If so, compile a list of everything that physicians use in the exam room. Keep an inventory. Inspect and stock the rooms daily. Remember, a physician will find supplies much faster if every exam room is set up exactly the same.

- Do physicians leave the exam room because information is missing that is needed for the patient encounter? If test results, hospital discharge summaries or consult notes are missing, implement a chart preview process.

- Do physicians fall behind schedule because they slip into their offices between visits to return a few telephone calls, and then start surfing the Internet and lose track of time? If so, convert an old supply closet or other small space near the exam rooms into a private workstation where physicians can quickly make telephone calls.

These and other common, time-consuming habits can easily be changed once you recognize the impact on physician productivity. For more tips on physician efficiency, see Chapter 7, "The Patient Encounter." Eliminate unnecessary steps, and physicians will spend more time doing what they love – seeing patients.

Maximizing your physician's time to increase patient volume

Let's say you anticipate that some of the patient flow improvements explained in this book will work for your practice. Before you go ahead with making those improvements, you may want to justify them by figuring the impact of increasing volume by, say, two visits a day, without adding any new physicians or staff.

Here are the basic figures for your practice:

- Fixed Cost: $10,000/month

- Physician Income: $20,000/month

- Revenue per Visit: $50

- Variable Cost per Visit: ($5)

- Contribution Margin per Visit: ($45)

- Current Number of Patient Visits: 667

Using these figures, add another 40 patient visits (that's about two per day in a typical 21-work day month). Don't worry right now about exactly how you will make it possible for your overworked physicians and staff to handle the additional patients – that's what we'll explore in the rest of this book.

Suppose we want to invest in new information technology, make other improvements, or increase the physician's income? Where do we find the additional revenue? In the case study, "Medical Practice Associates," we see what would happen if we could add 40 more visits per month by helping our physicians use time more efficiently.

Additional staffing can pay for itself if it improves the physician's productivity. Let's say there's a physician who has no medical assistants on staff and is able to see 15 patients a day. The fixed costs are $10,000 per month and the revenue per patient is $40. The physician needs to work 16 days each month to break even. The remaining four to nine workdays of the month are mostly profit (less other variable costs such as medical and administrative supplies).

Down the street is a physician who has a medical assistant and is able to see 30 patients a day. This physician also generates $40 per visit, but the fixed costs are $2,000 higher per month to pay for the medical assistant's salary and benefits. However, having the medical assistant makes it possible for the physician to cover the fixed costs in only 10 days. The last 10 to 15 workdays of the month are almost pure profit (less other variable costs such as medical and administrative supplies).

To generate an adequate volume of services, patient visits, RVUs – however your practice measures volume – and do it within an acceptable work period, the physician must be productive. An investment in additional resources – hiring the medical assistant – paid off well for the second physician in the prior example. A medical assistant may not double the physician's output but this resource can boost productivity significantly.

Medical Practice Associates increases revenue by adding volume

Medical Practice Associates needs $20,000 a month for physician income, plus $10,000 per month to cover fixed costs, for a total of $30,000 in monthly expenses. The practice receives $50 per visit, but has to spend $5 to pay the variable expenses of each visit. That leaves $45 to pay for fixed expenses per visit, plus what the physician wants to receive in income.

What if the physician could see two more patients a day, or 707 patients per month? The practice would now take in $31,815 in revenue ($45 per visit x 707 patients) each month. Since the fixed expenses are $10,000 per month, and the physician's desired income is $20,000 per month, subtracting it from the total net revenue leaves $1,815 to spend as we wish or to increase our physician's income.

Do the math:

Net Revenue per Visit ($45) x Patient Volume
(707 patients) = Total Revenue ($31,815)

Total Revenue ($31,815) - Total Fixed Cost
($30,000 per month) = $1,815

Over the course of a year, that additional revenue could support meaningful improvements to equipment, facility design or staffing for Medical Practice Associates.

Productive physicians are happier physicians (and so are their patients)

The less productive the physician is, the more the physician will have to work to produce the volume needed to cover the practice's fixed costs. The more inefficient the physician is, the greater the risk of burnout or bankruptcy, or both.

The productivity of a physician is directly related to time. Time, of course, is finite.

The physician only has so much time in which to produce volume. The more time the physician has to create the volume, the more revenue he or she can generate for the practice. It sounds pretty simple but don't forget that other simple concept: time is finite. The practice must consider allocating some of its resources to help its physicians use their practice time to create practice revenue. The three minutes it may take a physician to walk down two hallways of the practice to find a nurse to complete the patient visit and then to dig through a file drawer for a referral form is not time spent producing volume – it's just time wasted!

This isn't a chapter on staffing, but it should be pretty clear by now that a practice must consider allocating some resources on the fixed cost side (such as non-clinical staff time and information management equipment) to maximize the time of its revenue generators – its physicians.

The positive impact that certain fixed cost resources (staff, information technology, and so on) can have on the productivity of revenue-producing resources (physicians and midlevel providers) is why most medical practices have medical assistants do routine blood pressure checks, weigh-ins and certain other routine assessments when a patient checks in.

When expressed in terms of salary cost, the five or so minutes it takes a medical assistant to do these functions costs a fraction of the physician's five or so minutes. The physician could be generating revenue for the practice by spending that five or so minutes with another patient while the medical assistant prepares the next one. In coming chapters, I'll move beyond this basic timesaving step to look for other ways to make the best use of the time of physicians and the patients.

As you review the options and ideas explored in the next sections of this book, keep asking yourself, "Would this change improve the productivity of my physicians and midlevel providers?" If the answer is "yes," then the next question is, "How much fixed cost increase can I absorb to make this improvement work?" Finally, ask yourself if an increase to your fixed costs will generate at least the same amount of revenue. Unless there is a compelling reason to spend the money, don't do it. If new costs will not create similar or greater amount of offsetting revenue, then reconsider. The best costs to add are those that not only offset the costs, but also increase revenue above and beyond the costs.

Not all change is good

When do you absolutely never change a patient flow process? Leave things alone or look for more realistic solutions if the change will:

- Reduce physician productivity (you ask them to walk to the front office to retrieve all of their phone messages);

- Raise fixed costs more than the resulting physician productivity increases can cover (you ask Microsoft founder Bill Gates to personally design and install your new practice management system);

- Conflict with laws, regulations or contracts you have signed (you offer coupons for free services to Medicare patients);

- Compromise patient safety (you decide to make the patients draw their own blood); and

- Compromise patient convenience (you move to a much cheaper facility in a warehouse on the other side of town with limited parking).

Strategic considerations

There are a great many financial considerations in understanding how to make the best use of a physician's time, but there are many strategic considerations as well.

Yes, a physician's time is your most valuable asset, but simply increasing work hours should not be the sole solution. A good work/life balance with adequate personal time is the key to a happy – and productive – person. And, yes, I also recognize that increasing fixed and variable costs should be done carefully after considering all of the financial ramifications. But don't forget, patient service is always a consideration. Spending money to create better service is an investment, too – in creating loyal patients.

ADVANCED CONCEPT

Average Value of a Customer (AVC)

What is a patient worth to your practice? We've talked about the value of a physician's time but what happens if you forget about the patient's time? Unfortunately, many physicians and administrators do just that when they look at their already-full waiting rooms and do not consider the impact on operating costs from dissatisfied patients.

When a patient leaves before seeing the physician, the practice's costs for that patient's appointment – nurse's time, building space, utilities, equipment leases, and so on – do not walk out with that patient. All of that patient's cost to your practice's overhead stays behind. Those costs are subtracted from the practice income that, in many medical practices, is the physician's compensation. To illustrate to your physician the impact of losing patients, try calculating the average annual value of a patient.

This analysis should not replace a detailed cost accounting study, of course. Instead, it can be a quick and easy way to determine the "value" of each customer to your practice. Practices of all types can use their own data to develop similar measures for each of their physicians.

What's your AVC?

In order to calculate the Average Value of a Customer (AVC), NeuroAssociates had to first calculate its Average Revenue per Customer (ARC), shown in the table. To do this, NeuroAssociates divided its net collections (revenue) by its patient panel (unique patients) for the year. The result was a $240 ARC.

Don't confuse "patient visits" with patient panel in the "All Patients" column. A patient may visit a physician several times, but in column one, we are looking only for the value or revenue per patient, not per visit.

However, the values in the "Surgery Patients" column (column two) do represent unique visits since most patients make only one visit to the surgeon. If your practice's physicians often do more than one surgery or procedure per patient, then adjust column two accordingly.

The charges, revenue and volume number in the "Surgery Patients" column can be obtained by having the practice management system report all CPT codes for surgeries performed by the practice's surgeons.

Do the Math:

NeuroAssociates of Anytown

	All Patients	Surgery Patients
Total Gross Charges	$1,000,000	$500,000
Collections	$600,000	$300,000
Patient Panel	2,500	*
Patient Visits	550	*
ARC/Year	$240	$545
AVC/Year	$132	$245
		*not applicable

NeuroAssociates figured its ARC at $240. However, the ARC does not account for costs the practice must incur to serve its patients. NeuroAssociates applied its 45 percent overhead rate (total practice revenue divided by total fixed and variable practice costs) to the ARC, and determined that its AVC is $132. That is, each patient the practice served during the year contributed an average of $132 to the income of NeuroAssociates' physicians.

Since a smaller subset of NeuroAssociates' patients end up having surgery performed by the practice's physicians, the value of the higher revenue from this subset must be taken into account. Conducting the same ARC, AVC analysis of this subset produces a $545 ARC and $245 AVC.

If a physician member of NeuroAssociates saw an average of two fewer patients a week — either by cutting back on contact hours or having the patients walk out because they got tired of waiting — the impact would be a $12,140 loss in annual income (assuming a work year of 46 weeks). Assume that some of those patients would have needed surgery that the physician would have performed and the annual loss would amount to much more.

The average value of a patient of a primary care practice measures the "lifetime" value of that patient. Unlike specialists, primary care physicians are likely to have the customer (patient) over a period of years. They manage their patients' health until the patient moves out of town, changes insurance companies, becomes dissatisfied with the physician's service or leaves for other reasons. As described in the case study of NeuroAssociates, the value of the customer to a specialist is largely based on episodic care, not a long-term relationship. Given this assumption, you can calculate the AVC for a primary care physician using the following formula:

Average Value of a Customer

AVC = Cumulative retention rate *
(profit contribution margin - acquisition cost per customer - retention cost per customer)

Sample AVC of a family practitioner =

85% * [($50 contribution margin per visit * 4 visits per year * 15 years) -
($5 advertising and screening cost per patient) - ($.90 per visit per year * 4 visits * 15 years)

= $2,500

This analysis assumes the primary care practice's patients present an average of four times per year for 15 years. The practice's acquisition cost per patient is $5, while the practice spends $.90 per visit to retain the patient (beyond the cost of the office visit itself). The average value of a patient for this primary care practice is $2,500.

The principle of the average value of a customer (AVC) is the same for the specialist and the primary care physician. Because the primary care physician loses a "lifetime" of a patient versus an episode, the average value of their customers is higher. However, specialists have a lot more to lose in volume because their patients turn over much faster given the episodic nature of their practice. Either way, when you lose a patient, you lose income. Maintaining practice operations geared to patient service is not only valuable to your patients, it is valuable to you...in real dollars.

New physicians

Has this ever happened in your practice? You hire a new physician but find months later that the new physician books just 10 patients a day – too few to cover his salary and overhead.

Try lending your new physicians a hand. Track performance monthly and look for ways to help them become successes in your practice. Here's how:

Check the new physician's schedule each month. Compare time-to-next-available-appointment averages for new and established physicians in your practice. Is the new physician's average time to next appointment much longer than that of established physicians? The new physician's scheduling template may be to blame. The template may have too many slots reserved for established patient slots that go unfilled. For the first two years at a minimum, ask new physicians to be very flexible with appointment types so they can build their active patient panel. See Chapter 4, "Scheduling," for additional discussion of the scheduling template problem.

Count the number of new patient appointments each month. Compare them to the total number of appointments scheduled. Plot this ratio on a graph, month after month. The number of new patient visits should stay steady or, better, it should grow each month.

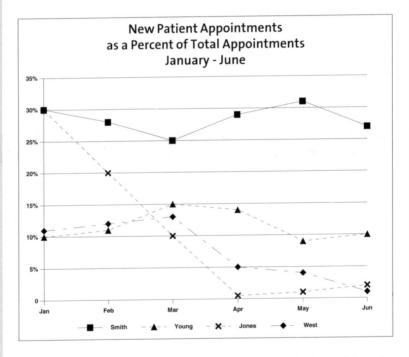

Dr. Jones is experiencing a rapid decline in his new patient appointments as a percent of his total appointments. If his volume of encounters remains the same, he will soon experience a decline in revenue. If he is a surgeon or a proceduralist, revenue will fall dramatically.

If the average number of new patient appointments per month falls, it may be a sign that new patients — or the physicians who refer them — are not interested in the new physician. Or it might indicate a fault in the scheduling process, such as schedulers forgetting to send new patients to the new physician. It could even be caused by your practice's internal politics – a more established physician has told schedulers to keep sending new patients to her.

Promote the new physician. Hold an open house, a reception for referring physicians, and place an advertisement in the local paper to promote the new physician's arrival in the practice. If the new physician is replacing another physician, send an informational mailing to patients who might be reassigned to the new physician. And don't forget to include the new physician's name in your telephone directory ad and on your Web site. Make sure that the new physician is credentialed and signed up with all of your insurance plans as soon as possible; ask her to sign the paperwork the same day that she signs her employment contract.

Set expectations. A young physician might not know how many patients he should be able to see in a day. Set very clear goals and offer him real-world advice on how to meet them.

New physicians can help your practice tremendously. Monitoring their progress can help you and them!

Going solo

More and more physicians, frustrated by high overhead, staff squabbles, and the bureaucracy that often comes with large practices, are considering solo practice. The model of these solo practice is different than years past – solo physicians are often looking to cut back staff or eliminate staff altogether. How? They are harnessing technology to streamline workflow, outsourcing some functions, and doing more of the work themselves. It can be a realistic vision but only for physicians with realistic expectations.

Consider these factors before going solo:

A physician certainly can get along with few or even no staff. She can check in patients, room them, and listen for the phone to ring. After clinic or between patients, she can submit claims and call insurance companies with any questions. That said, be aware of the demands of filling out forms, answering telephones, negotiating insurance contracts, submitting claims, following up on claims denials, inventorying supplies and so on. It can be exhausting – and complex. It's critical to have trusted advisers or an excellent grasp on key financial and other performance indicators to make sure your practice is staying on the right track.

With fewer staff, a solo physician can lower her revenue expectations without a drop in income. If she's spending $100,000 less in staff, for example, then she can reduce her revenue by $100,000 without decreasing her income. Simply put, the physician doesn't have to see as many patients to make the practice work. However, although having few or no staff greatly reduces overhead, there are many other expenses to running a medical practice – malpractice and other insurance, supplies, equipment, office space, taxes, marketing and so on. Don't forget that going solo doesn't mean eliminating the entire overhead of a practice.

Although the physician can see fewer patients, sometimes this can backfire. Since physicians are notoriously bad at saying "no," controlling demand can be a difficult task. If you hear yourself saying, "oh, I'll just squeeze in a few more patients..." everyday, you may soon find yourself overwhelmed with the demands of seeing patients – and taking care of all of the administrative issues that result. Consider limiting your patient panel by negotiating participation agreements with only certain insurance companies to help control demand.

Invest in technology – early. Start off your practice with an electronic medical record and automate as much of your workflow as possible. It's much easier to start with a "paperless" office than it is to transition into one.

Shedding staff can relieve an incredible emotional burden on physicians who simply don't like to handle conflict or manage people. Some physicians enjoy the reduced complexity and lower overhead of the solo operation. They are comfortable spending part of the day doing nonmedical tasks. And, when faced with repetitive clerical tasks, they try not to say, "I didn't go to medical school to do *this*." Instead, they like the diversity — and the simplicity — of it all.

Chapter 3

TELEPHONES

Key Chapter Lessons

> Familiarize yourself with key telephone concepts

> Calculate your "Telephone IQ"

> Develop a thorough analysis of your current system and future needs

> Learn about valuable telephone reports

> Recognize steps to change telephone demand

> Create a "mystery telephone patient survey"

> Understand the pros and cons of telephony applications for your practice

> Find tips for voice mail, ACDs (automatic call distributors), and auto attendants

> Recognize steps to select or change your telephone system

> Learn about staffing your telephones – and what to watch out for

Advanced Concepts

> HIPAA and your telephone

Learn to handle telephones; or they will handle you!

There are many ways to improve the physician's use of time and make patients happy but, maybe, the most important influence on how a patient moves through a practice is that low-tech, often-overlooked tool – the telephone.

Before patients come in for appointments, they generally call. That's your first opportunity to impress them with good, efficient service – and get the data that make life easy for your physicians.

The telephone is your friend, honest!

What's happening with the telephones in your practice? Do patients complain about busy signals or long hold times? Do referring physicians complain that they can never get through? Do staff members spend too much time chasing down answers to questions from callers who just want to renew routine prescriptions or get test results? If so, then your telephone system and how you use it both need an overhaul.

Telephone demand is what you make it

When telephones demand more staff time or patients can't get through, the traditional solution has been to add more telephone lines, new equipment, and/or another telephone operator. These steps may be necessary but there may be other options to look to before devoting more resources to these traditional solutions to telephone problems. For example, consider changing how you handle scheduling, prescription renewals, referrals and other processes to reduce tele-phone demand. Maybe your practice is unintentionally causing many of its current telephone problems.

Take a few minutes to assess the general state of the telephone system in your practice by completing the "What's Your Telephone IQ?" test on pages 36 to 37. Did you score above 75? If so, keep everything just as it is. You also have permission to skip this chapter and consider moonlighting as a telecommunications consultant because your practice is among the very few that have no major telephone issues.

For the rest of the world, please read on to learn how to assess your telephone system and discover ways to change the processes that may be artificially stimulating high telephone demand.

Changing telephone demand

❑ Track call volume.

❑ Do mystery shopper surveys and review results.

❑ Gather data from telephone system and/or by observation.

❑ Ask staff to collect data on inbound call topics.

❑ Analyze outbound calls to find patterns.

❑ Analyze the current telephone system's pluses and minuses.

Inefficient telephones cost money

What are the consequences of having an inefficient telephone system? Consider this: the telephone is your physicians' main link to the outside world. Without it, patients don't get scheduled, referrals are not made or received, patient triage is delayed or doesn't happen, after-hours questions from patients don't get handled, prescriptions don't get renewed, claims can't be followed up, and so on. With all of this at stake, why do so many medical practices turn this vital lifeline over to the lowest paid, least trained and, often, least experienced employee?

WORSHEET

What is Your Telephone IQ?

Directions: Read through each question carefully. Being as honest as you can, indicate the appropriate evaluation as described below:

5 = Excellent – Keep as is
4 = Above average – Opportunities still exist
3 = Average – Improvements need to be made
2 = Fair – Needs attention
1 = Poor – Below acceptable standards for our practice

When you finish, consider areas you marked 1 or 2 and decide how and when to improve. If you don't know the answers to the questions, be sure to find out the answer!

_____ 1. The number of incoming lines is adequate to handle both peak and low times.

_____ 2. Callers are not kept on hold for more than two minutes.

_____ 3. We ask every caller's permission before putting him or her on hold.

_____ 4. Everyone in the practice who answers the telephone uses his or her name and the practice's name.

_____ 5. Specific backup personnel are scheduled so the telephones are answered promptly.

_____ 6. Everyone has been trained thoroughly on the telephone equipment.

_____ 7. We have up-to-date equipment with the latest time-saving features.

_____ 8. Periodic telephone training is provided to fine-tune telephone skills.

_____ 9. Callers don't complain about busy signals when they call our practice.

_____ 10. Callers don't complain about being put on hold excessively.

_____ 11. Callers are not disconnected when we transfer calls.

_____ 12. Callers don't complain about the complexity of the system.

_____ 13. The telephones are always covered (during regular working hours).

_____ 14. All calls are answered by the third ring.

_____ 15. Voice mail messages are kept current, are helpful, and sound pleasant and friendly.

_____ 16. Callers don't complain that their messages go unanswered.

_____ TOTAL

76-80 = You are the Gold Standard! Congratulations.

60-75 = Opportunities still exist. Explore staffing, system and functional changes.

45-59 = Start making changes to improve the system and process.

<45 = Get right on it! Your patients and referring physicians need you to make improvements so that they can access your practice.

Modified from work of ©University Physicians, Inc., Baltimore, MD, 2003. Used with permission.

Pay attention to workers' needs

❑ Start enhancing your telephone system by improving working conditions for your telephone operators. Discuss equipment needs with staff. Do they need hands-free headsets? Better chairs? You may avoid future worker's compensation claims, and you will gain the operators' buy-in to assist with other practice duties.

A new telephone system

With 10 surgeons in three specialties, nearly 40 employees and a large patient base, we get a huge number of telephone calls daily. We had never taken the time to audit our actual volume by using a flow sheet highlighting call volume patterns. However, when our operations consultant spent a week with us conducting an audit of this and other areas, the results were highly illuminating. We realized staffing patterns had to change and the case for buying a new telephone system was greatly enhanced.

Our previous system was nearly 15 years old – no voice mail, no selective paging, and no hands-free operations – well, you get the picture. A new state of the art system was installed coupled with T1 line technology. DID (direct inward dialing) now takes much of the load off the switchboard; voice mail allows for faster triaging of telephone calls; paging is a programmable, hands-free operation; and conferencing and programmed speed dialing are available on every telephone. What a difference this new technology has made in the ease, efficiency, and speed of handling telephone calls.

Ken Hertz, Administrator, MacArthur Surgical Clinic, Alexandria, LA

E-mail and online links that can handle these processes are not yet widespread enough to allow you to ignore the problems you are having with your telephones today.

Instead of hiring extra staff, adding more telephone lines or waiting for new technology to make the problem go away, let's look at ways to redesign patient flow processes so that demand for the telephone is actually reduced instead of simply redirected. The demands that cannot be eliminated can be shifted to the most appropriate stage of the patient flow process and to the most appropriate person.

Warning: These time- and money-saving ideas to change your telephone demand may involve changing resource allocations, altering telephone triage systems, implementing new technologies, relearning current technologies, and changing staff responsibilities.

Tracking call volumes

Most automated telephone systems can produce reports that show the volume of calls that came in each hour, day or week, as well as how many rings before the call was answered, the time callers waited on hold, and how many calls were abandoned. If you aren't sure whether or not your current automated telephone system can produce these reports, contact your vendor or dig up your system's instruction manual and read it. Newer systems should be able to produce these reports with very little hassle. Ask the vendor how you can get the reports. You may need special software.

When buying your next telephone system, don't consider one that doesn't put reporting capabilities at your fingertips.

In addition to the number of calls processed per hour and by which operator, it is important to know your practice's call abandonment rate. In other words, how often are incoming calls not processed?

Why are these reports so important? Because they are the first place to look when trying to solve telephone issues. These reports can tell you if your attempts to change telephone demand are working.

Telephone system reports

✓ Time on hold report
✓ Time of day report
✓ Calls per day report
✓ Number of calls processed
✓ Amount of time on each call
✓ Abandonment rate

Track inbound calls first

If your telephone system cannot produce reports (or you wish to supplement them), you can track the inbound calls manually. Understanding the nature of inbound calls will help the telephone system assessment process.

Give a tracking sheet to the practice's operators and other staff assigned to handle inbound patient calls. Ask them to track the calls they receive within each hour block for a minimum of three consecutive days. Remind the call trackers each morning and several times throughout the day. It may take a couple of attempts to get a complete enough record. Although you are not looking for statistical perfection, it's important not to underestimate the volume of inbound calls or miss an important category.

To make the job easier, provide a form that allows call trackers to check off the most common topics. Be sure to that your call trackers mark any calls that are repeat calls – that is, the caller has called once (or more times) previously without getting resolution to his or her question. To do this, ask call trackers to make a special mark on the log whenever the patient indicates that they have already called about the issue.

Inbound Call Tracking Form

Instructions: Place a slash mark "|" for each call. If the patient calls BACK, place a DOT on the slash mark "|".

Name: ─────────────────────────────

Date: ─────────────────────────────

Phone Extension: ─────────────────────────

	Prescriptions	Scheduling	Billing	Referrals	Test Results	Nurse/Physician	Other	TOTAL
8 to 9								
9 to 10								
10 to 11								
11 to 12								
12 to 1								
1 to 2								
2 to 3								
3 to 4								
4 to 5								

The value of this exercise is that you might learn, for example, that 30 percent of your incoming calls concern laboratory results, 10 percent are for prescription refills, and five percent are for directions to your new satellite clinic.

Of course, you'll want this survey information to be gathered only at the point of the practice's first live contact with the patient's inbound call. Placing these survey forms at back office telephones could result in transferred calls being counted two or more times, depending on how many times the patient is transferred.

After you've looked at the categories, calculate the percentage of the total calls that were repeat calls. In many practices, as many as 30 percent of the total incoming calls are repeat calls.

...you're having telephone problems when...

...the number of walk-in patients starts increasing. This can occur when patients who feel they have pressing problems cannot get through to the scheduling desk or to anyone who can triage their questions. Frustrated by your telephone tie-ups, these patients will show up unannounced (and probably get more frustrated if your practice hasn't taken action on the tips in Chapter 4, "Scheduling"), or worse, find someplace else to go.

No matter how you accomplish it, make sure you know why your patients are calling before making significant changes to any processes. You may discover inadequacies in other processes such as patient education, prescription refills, test result notification, referrals, or scheduling. Areas in which there are a high percent of repeat calls are prime opportunities to improve your practice. Target those areas first for your performance improvement initiatives.

Distribute the results of your incoming call analysis and engage staff and physicians in discussions of what might be sparking these patterns. Further analysis may show that a physician is telling patients to call back the following day to get their laboratory test results. Or, you may discover that you need to do a better job of promoting your new clinic's location or instructing patients to call their pharmacy, not the medical practice, for routine refills.

Sample Results Telephone Analysis

Type of Call	Total	% Repeat
RX	32	28.1%
Scheduling	30	0.0%
Test Results	35	2.9%
Nurse/Phys	45	33.3%
Billing/Referral	12	33.3%
Other	16	0.0%
TOTAL	170	26.5%

Repeat calls are 26.5 percent of incoming volume.

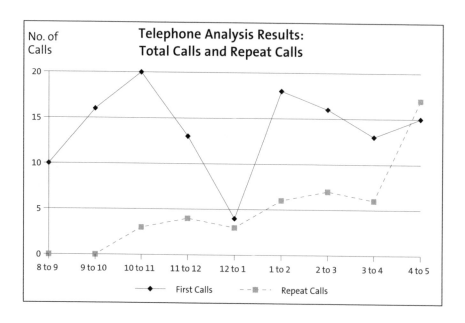

Informed staff reduces risk

- Make sure administrative staff know basic medical terminology. Everyone whose duties include answering a telephone must be able to correctly spell important medical terms that describe chief complaints, diagnoses, medications, etc. Indecipherable messages force you to call back patients, pharmacies, laboratories or other physicians to figure out what they said. That's just more work for you.

- Make sure that any staff member who would ever answer your telephones – even a medical records clerk working after hours – recognizes patient emergencies and has guidelines to handle extenuating circumstances with referring physicians. I'm not suggesting that the records clerk become your triage nurse, but you never know who will be around when a crisis occurs. An informed staff means an efficient office. It's good risk management and good patient service.

Call volume

- ❑ Standard expectation for primary care: 100 to 200 calls per physician per day

- ❑ Standard expectation for specialists: 75 to 125 calls per physician per day

Your call volume may fall out of these ranges depending on the maturity of your practice, the needs of your patients, and your practice's success in managing telephone demand.

Mystery patient survey

To supplement your internal analyses, try a mystery patient survey. Ask a friend or colleague to call your practice and note how often they get busy signals, how long they wait on hold, what they hear while on hold, and their impressions of the courtesy of the staff answering the telephones (who should not be told that the survey is being conducted).

If possible, have the surveyors attempt to call the practice during each hour block, that is, 8:00 to 9:00 a.m., 9:00 to 10:00 a.m., etc. You may be surprised – and not always pleasantly – by what happens when people call in during the lunch hour, immediately after the practice opens in the morning, or just before closing. The mystery telephone patient survey will not give you all the answers you need to fully assess your telephone system, but it will give more credibility to anecdotal information you may hear from patients. Mystery telephone patient survey reports can be combined with reports produced by your telephone system and with other observations to give a clearer picture of what's going right and/or wrong with your telephone system.

The Mystery Telephone Patient Survey

Pick one of these sample questions:

1. Can you give me directions to your office?
2. Can you tell me something about Dr. _____?
3. Do you accept _____ insurance?
4. How long would I have to wait to get a physical exam with Dr. _____?

Practice: _____   Caller: _____

Call Date: _____   Call time: _____

❏ Exceeds standards ❏ Meets Standards ❏ Does not meet standards

Number of rings: ❏ 1   ❏ 2   ❏ 3   ❏ More than 4

Courtesy of person answering telephone
❏ Very pleasant   ❏ Pleasant   ❏ Rude or hurried

Did the person answering the telephone give you his or her name?
❏ Gave name clearly   ❏ Gave name   ❏ Did not give name

Did the person answering the telephone give you the practice's name?
❏ Gave name clearly   ❏ Gave name   ❏ Did not give name

Did you get put on hold?
❏ Never put on hold
❏ Briefly put on hold after being asked if ok
❏ Put on hold without being asked

If you were put on hold, how long did you wait?
❏ Less than 30 seconds   ❏ 30 to 90 seconds
❏ More than 90 seconds

Level of knowledge of person answering telephone
❏ Extremely knowledgeable; gave complete, correct information immediately
❏ Knowledgeable; gave correct information
❏ Gave incorrect information

Level of concern of person answering telephone
❏ Demonstrated high level of genuine interest in caller
❏ Demonstrated interest in caller
❏ Demonstrated little or no interest in caller

Were you transferred to another individual who ultimately answered your question?
❏ Not transferred; call handled by first person
❏ Transferred once to correct person with appropriate explanation
❏ Transferred more than once, transferred to wrong person or transferred without appropriate explanation

Was a message taken for someone to call you back?
❏ Message not taken; call handled by first person
❏ Message taken appropriately; received call back in specified time
❏ Message taken inappropriately; call not returned in specified time

Courtesy of person answering question
❏ Very pleasant   ❏ Pleasant   ❏ Rude or hurried

Did person answering the question give his or her name?
❏ Gave name clearly   ❏ Gave name   ❏ Did not give name

Did you get put on hold by the person who answered the question?
❏ Never put on hold
❏ Briefly put on hold after being asked if ok
❏ Put on hold without being asked

If put on hold by this person, how long did you wait?
❏ Less than 30 seconds   ❏ 30 to 90 seconds
❏ More than 90 seconds

Knowledge of person answering question
❏ Extremely knowledgeable; gave complete, correct information immediately
❏ Knowledgeable; gave correct information
❏ Gave incorrect information

Level of concern of person answering question
❏ Demonstrated high level of genuine interest in caller
❏ Demonstrated interest in caller
❏ Demonstrated little or no interest in caller

Comments to support ratings exceeding or not meeting standards:
_____

Outbound calls can be time wasters

After organizing your internal call reports, staff observations about incoming calls, and the results of your mystery patient survey, analyze outbound calls to find patterns. A form similar to that used for inbound calls may help. Just don't confuse staff by doing the inbound and outbound surveys at the same time – unless the inbound calls are received by a different individual (e.g., telephone operator) than the one who places outbound calls (e.g., triage nurse). In this case, give the inbound tracking form to the telephone operator and the outbound form to the nurse.

If it seems that the percentages of outbound calls by topic match up with those of inbound calls, then there may be some room for improvement in the process related to that topic. For example, a high volume of inbound and outbound calls dealing with laboratory results may indicate that your staff and patients are spending too much time playing telephone tag when other, simpler communications solutions might work.

No matter what measurement tool you have used, it is more than likely that you've concluded that performance improvement is needed, if not essential. There are several ways to change the processes that can spur telephone demand. The following sections spotlight strategies to help you improve performance.

Stop playing "pass the caller"

Does this happen in your practice? The receptionist transfers a patient's call to the scheduler, the scheduler cannot determine if the patient is sick enough to deserve one of the practice's precious few slots for acute appointments, the patient is transferred to the nurse, the nurse puts the patient on hold to consult with the physician, and, finally, the patient is transferred back to the scheduler. The accumulated time for all of these transfers? Up to 30 minutes. The amount of value-added time to the medical practice? Maybe, 3 minutes. The amount of frustration to the patient: impossible to estimate.

The lesson of this all-too-frequent game of transfer tag is that you must develop internal processes to combine tasks and limit telephone transfers. Don't waste your patients' time. Don't tie up your telephone lines so other patients can't call for appointments. Route callers to staff who can get the entire job done.

Allowing the appropriate staff to get the job done without all of the transfers is perhaps the greatest asset that an electronic medical record can offer to your operations. With the patient's information close at hand, the needs of many callers – from patients to referring physicians – can be handled more expeditiously. If you implement an electronic medical record, make sure that you are taking advantage of your practice's ability to get the job done, thereby eliminating the many inefficiencies of playing "pass the caller."

Avoid unnecessary repeat calls

If you don't have the ability to process the calls as they come in, set a policy in your practice regarding a timeframe for calling patients, referring physicians and other callers back. I recommend no more than two hours because it is courteous to patients who are often sitting by the phone waiting for your call. If you cannot resolve the patient's question within two hours, call the patient back to inform him about the status of your response. This will avoid having the caller call back – again and again – asking the same question. This ties up staff time unnecessarily and fosters caller frustration and even anger.

Scheduling: decentralize it

How many calls does your triage nurse answer per hour? How many of those calls end up with the patient needing an appointment scheduled?

More than likely your triage nurse is not trained to schedule appointments. No wonder your scheduling staff is so busy. No wonder patients are upset: they likely had to wade through a telephone tree, wait on hold to get to the triage nurse, then wait on hold again to get an appointment. By training whoever handles triage to also schedule patients, you shift that demand away from other staff. More important, you score points for good customer service.

Don't deflect demand

Consider the time your practice spends on deflecting appointment demand. The role of many triage nurses is to analyze the acuity of patients to determine if they need appointments. That is, the patients who are really sick will receive same-day appointments, while most other patients are deflected. These patients are scheduled to come in at a future date because there are no appointments immediately available. The resources expended in demand deflection are tremendous, and many medical practices are re-engineering their appointment schedules to create more access...and to reduce this cost, which adds no value. (See Chapter 4, "Scheduling," for more information.)

Checkout: the place to schedule all follow-up visits

If there are procedural, software, hardware, or other obstacles that prevent patients from scheduling follow-up visits at checkout, then work hard to remove them. You will only aggravate your patients by making them walk to another desk to wait or, worse, force them to call back in to an already overloaded telephone system.

Scheduling follow-up visits at checkout will eliminate many but not all such inbound calls. It is inevitable that some patients will realize later on that they have a conflict with the appointment date.

Create appointment templates that cover a minimum of three months. Although practices are moving towards fast access, there will always be a need to schedule certain follow-up appointments for patients. Other patients may need to plan office visits around work hours, vacations, and other commitments.

...telephone processes need work when...

... your scheduling system creates more incoming calls. At the checkout counter with my 4-month-old son, I asked if I could schedule his next well-baby visit, only eight weeks away. I'm sorry," she said. "We can only schedule appointments through the end of the month." Her next words were – you guessed it! – "just give us a call." The result? Saving the 30 seconds or less it would take to schedule my appointment on the spot became several minutes of staff and my time next month.

Rescheduling: Learn how to say "no"

A physician changes clinic hours. Your staff goes into high gear to quickly contact patients to reschedule appointments. Of course, you never seem to get most patients on the telephone on the first try, so you and your staff must leave messages on answering machines or in voice-mail boxes or try calling alternate telephone numbers. And, of course, every one of those patients has to call back to reschedule.

Don't let physicians create all of this work. Wise medical practices ask physicians to establish clinic schedules and stick to them. Limit rescheduling to emergencies.

Reminders can reduce telephone demand

How else can you reduce telephone call volumes? Try sending out reminders to patients four to five days in advance of their appointments, or calling patients two days in advance. Yes, it will increase your costs. But that small additional cost will likely be offset by a great savings in the amount of time that staff must spend handling incoming calls from patients who can't recall the exact time or day of their appointment. It may also produce cost-savings by reducing no-shows or late arrivals.

Many practices are automating reminder telephone calls to patients. These systems can work well and can be integrated into many new practice management systems. Just make sure the calls are friendly sounding and do not breach patient confidentiality; that is, the automated message must not say what complaint the appointment is for. (See Advanced Concepts, "HIPAA and your telephones" for more information about reminders.)

Let schedulers schedule

Too many practices do not allow their schedulers to schedule. You can tell these practices almost at a glance. They are the ones where the staff answering telephones must constantly leave their workstations, and hunt down physicians, nurses or other physicians for permission to schedule an appointment. Just one or two physicians in the practice who insist on approving all appointments in advance can cost dearly in terms of staff time.

When schedulers have to continually ask permission to do their jobs, patients are left on hold and incoming lines are tied up. Or, worse, schedulers must play a completely unnecessary game of telephone tag with patients.

If you're a subspecialty practice with an appropriate need to screen appointments, see the Advanced Concept on preappointment screening in Chapter 4, "Scheduling," for more information.

Prescriptions

Most encounters with a physician include a medication – an initial prescription, a change of medication, or a refill. There are several steps that you can take to better handle prescriptions – and consequently, reduce your telephone calls.

Practices that have implemented prescription refill lines with voice-mail boxes often receive messages like this: "This is Mary Smith. I need my 'little blue pills' refilled." Thus begins another game of telephone tag as the nurse tries to figure out who Mary Smith is, how to contact her for more information, and what the "little blue pills" are.

Ask your patients to call their pharmacies for refills. Ask pharmacists to fax the requests to you for approval. Better still, establish a secure electronic interface with local pharmacies or utilize automated prescription software. Many large drug store chains offer these options because they want your patients' business. Whatever solution you choose will mean that your staff and the pharmacy's staff spend less time waiting on hold for refill approvals. Streamlining this communication link also means you will get the documentation you need for the patient's medical record. If it's not automatically downloaded to your electronic medical record, remember to write the refill request or questions from the pharmacy on an adhesive label and attach to the patient's record so that you don't have to transcribe it again.

Some patients will still call about refills, so create a voice-mail box in your telephone system with prompts for them to leave requests and questions. Set up protocols about how your staff will handle those requests and questions. Prescriptions must be refilled promptly or the patient must be advised why not as soon as possible. You don't want patients or pharmacists to feel like their requests are going into a black box.

Your prescription writing protocols also can add to telephone overload. Residency clinics, for example, often get more telephone calls for prescription refills than do private practices. The reason is that residency clinics typically write prescriptions for a shorter cycle. Of course, maintaining your standard of care is more important than boosting telephone efficiency but there are many valid reasons to evaluate prescribing protocols annually to see if they are up to date.

What one question asked during a patient's office visit can help reduce your volume of prescription refill calls? The question is, "do you need any prescription refilled today?" Too many times, a refill call comes from the patient who was in the office just the week before. Try printing paper tablets with the heading: "Refills I Need to Discuss with my Doctor Today." Leave the tablets and pencils around the reception area or in each exam room. Make the refill question part of the rooming process.

To avoid callbacks from pharmacies, scrutinize the legibility of your physician's handwriting. Often, illegible handwriting prompts a phone call from the pharmacist to clarify the medication, dosage or other instructions. Automated prescription software will eliminate these phone calls by printing prescriptions and/or transmitting them directly to the pharmacy.

Manage patient-to-physician calls better

"I only want to talk to my doctor." Ever heard a patient say that? If you are hearing it a lot, then it's time to consider taking a team approach to health care delivery. Patients who consistently see one clinical assistant or nurse each time they visit their doctor are much more likely to open up to this individual. Your verbal support for that assistant is critical. Tell the patient that the assistant is an important member of your "team." Reinforce your assistants' credibility by printing business cards for them. It's a small investment that creates greater credibility, and better patient access.

Follow-up calls

Historically, surgical practices would always place a phone call to their patients on the day following discharge. This activity still occurs, but it is no longer common practice. In addition to leaving an indelible impression on the patient, these calls can also have a positive impact on practice operations.

Proactively calling a patient prevents medical problems from getting complicated. Complications drive up phone calls, medication requests and office visits, as well as the obvious negative impact on the patient's care.

If you're a surgical practice or perform procedures, try calling your patients one or two days after the service. Review medical instructions, evaluate the patient's improvement, adjust medications if appropriate, and reinforce discharge instructions. In addition to preventing future phone calls, this single phone call may be your best marketing technique – and it helps your patients get better faster.

Take messages that stick

Practices routinely receive hundreds of phone messages each day. Many of these messages need to be recorded because they are of a clinical nature and concern the management of the patient's care. Instead of taking the message on a piece of paper that will be thrown away and later transcribing the message into its permanent location, write the message only once. By collapsing these two processes into one, you'll save staff time that you're now dedicating to an unnecessary activity.

Taking messages on labels is a very simple concept. Whoever takes a patient message concerning a clinically related question should write that message on a label that can be applied to the appropriate page in the patient's chart. Notes of calls handled by triage nurses should be put on labels that can be quickly attached to the official patient record.

Do the same for handling communications from referring physicians.

An idea for practices wanting a "low tech" solution is to convert phone messages to e-mails or e-mail attachments. Route the message to the e-mail box belonging to the person who should receive and respond to the message. Print the e-mail as documentation, or electronically attach it to the patient's account.

If you have an electronic medical record, type messages directly into the system instead of having to write and then subsequently type the information.

Managing test results

Many medical practices still tell patients: "If you don't hear anything from us, everything is okay." That may make it easy on the staff but it is hardly considerate of the patient. Patients may want to know their exact cholesterol levels, how they compare to last year's test, and what the physician thinks about it. Often, keeping patients in the dark will just spur them to call in to get the information, which can tie up your staff.

One way to avoid tying up your staff is to implement an automated test results retrieval program. The nurse or physician records the information in a special voice-mail box set up just for the patient. The patient receives a phone number and personal identification number to access the box. This may avoid telephone tag, but be sure to evaluate its costs and test the user-friendliness of the system.

Why not be proactive and make test results part of the patient education function? Design your own form or brochure or use one provided by your specialty society to explain common test results. Mailing out this information out with test results will cost a few extra cents and use a little more staff time, but it won't cost nearly as much as the time you probably spend now to dig out test results and find a clinician to explain them when patients call in with questions.

Be realistic about the timing of test results. Establish your patients' expectations when they leave the exam room. Give yourself some wiggle room. If it usually takes three days to get the result of a MRI, then tell the patient it will likely be four days. If a test result is abnormal, you – and the patient – will likely hear of it long before the fourth day. If you promise four days but call earlier, then the patient is delighted with your service.

Ask your patients how they want to receive test results. The most common methods of delivery are voice mail, answering machine, e-mail, letter, or no delivery at all (if results are normal). Create a form for your practice to ask this question of all patients. Flag patients' records to show their preferences and adhere to their desires.

If you don't have a patient-directed protocol established or don't want to manage a multi-faceted reporting system, the most efficient way to report test results is to try once to contact the patient. If unsuccessful, then follow up with a confidential letter.

Don't leave test results in a voice-mail box or e-mail unless you have written permission to do so, *and* the results are normal. If you don't reach the patient or don't have permission to leave a message, mail the results in a confidential manner immediately following that call, rather than waiting a day and calling back. This process allows you to report information as you are processing the work, prevents the vicious cycle of callbacks, and lets you immediately re-file the chart.

Unless there are extenuating circumstances, never give patients abnormal test results via a telephone message or letter. This news should be delivered in person or when you are able to talk with them on the telephone.

Is your communication with other physicians efficient? Or is it creating more work? Reduce to a single notification the communication of test results between your practice and other physicians. Some ancillary or specialty service providers will send their test results or conclusions to you by e-mail with a follow up telephone call. Then, they will send you a fax of the results and follow that up by mailing you a hard copy. Your staff might receive a patient's test results several times over. If this duplication creates a paperwork or communication problem, work with your laboratories and other providers to streamline their communications into one — and only one — mode.

Frustrated by the inability to deliver results in a patient-friendly manner, some practices now just schedule a return visit to review the results. The appointment is scheduled a couple of days after the results are expected back. This procedure is very prevalent when a more serious test is ordered, such as a biopsy.

(For more information on managing test results, see Chapter 8, "Checkout.")

STEPS
TO GET YOU THERE

Reduce call volumes for test results

1. Transmitting results to patients in a confidential letter or secure Internet correspondence (or Web look-up)

2. Allowing patients to call into a confidential, password-controlled voice-mail box set up just for them

3. Increasing the amount and quality of patient education that accompanies test results to try and answer common questions

Reduce unnecessary clinical calls

Looking for ways to reduce unnecessary follow-up telephone calls from patients without alienating them? Do a better job of anticipating — and answering — patients' questions before they leave the office.

Rural physicians and doctors who cover call on weekends or evenings are not the only ones who spend too much time answering telephone calls about non-urgent clinical questions. Studies show that up to half of the calls a medical practice receives about clinical matters come from patients who were just seen in the office. Many times, these patients ask for information they should have received – and probably did receive – during a recent office visit.

Use the sample Incoming Clinical Calls Log to track incoming clinical telephone calls for several weeks. The information from this log will help you improve patient-physician communications, reduce the volume of incoming clinical telephone calls to your practice, and enhance patient education.

It may seem impossible to ask your clinical staff to spend more time teaching patients but improving in-office written and verbal communications will reduce incoming call volume. You could see the results in just a few weeks. Your patients will be better educated and more medically compliant, and your practice will operate more efficiently.

Incoming Clinical Calls Log

Date	Nurse initials	Time	Date of previous appt (ask patient or look up)	Was the patient's appt within the last week? (Y/N)	Reason for call (Summary)

Follow these steps for best results:

1. Ask everyone in your practice who handles clinical calls to use the Incoming Clinical Calls Log.

2. Record the general purpose of each patient's call, the date of the call, and the date of his or her last appointment. Look this up at the end of the day if you don't have time to do it as the calls are coming in.

3. Keep the logs for a few weeks, then review the entries in the "Reason for Call (Summary)" column. Group the frequently asked questions into basic categories. For example, a surgical practice may be able to group patient questions into:

   - Preoperative instructions: "Can I take a Tylenol the day before surgery?"

   - Postoperative wound care: "What do I do if it's been three days since the surgery and the site is still tender?"

   - Logistics: "What time should I be at the hospital?"

   - General questions: "Can I drink a beer with this medication?"

4. Count the questions in each category.

5. Note the time elapsed since the patient's last appointment and highlight those received within one week of the patient's last appointment.

6. Review the results with the physicians and nurses. Look for patterns. Note which categories had the most questions and which questions are asked most often.

7. Discuss how your practice can proactively educate your patients about the frequently cited categories and pay particular attention to the questions asked by patients who were just seen in the office.

8. Perform the call logging exercise biannually and look for other trends.

9. Seek solutions such as:

   - Asking the patient during or at the end of the appointment if he has questions about the visit and his care;

   - Developing a "Q&A" for the diagnoses or services provided most frequently to your patients;

   - Purchasing or developing videos or brochures that describe the treatment plans your physicians use most often;

   - Offering patients a handout with Web sites, support groups, or other resources that you recommend;

   - Proactively addressing side effects of medications, procedures, or treatments; and

   - Developing an action plan for the patient regarding the treatment and present it to the patient in a notebook that includes a log for the patient to use to record details about his or her care.

What time is your callback?

Schedule patients for their telephone callbacks with physicians or nurses. This will maximize the physician's or nurse's time and improve their relationship with patients. Plus it helps everybody avoid the annoying game of telephone tag.

Billing and referrals

How can you reduce telephone calls from patients with billing questions? Review your billing statements. Can you understand them? If you can't, rest assured that your patients can't either. Revising statements for better clarity will reduce the number of telephone calls to billing staff.

Give your billing and referral department their own phone numbers. Print those numbers on billing statements so patients can call them directly. Set up an e-mail account (billing@yourpractice name.com) to improve access to your billing staff.

Anticipate general information requests

The time that your staff spends on the telephone with new patients who need directions to the clinic can be reduced somewhat by sending out a "welcome to our practice" packet to all new patients before their first appointment. Send packets to all returning patients when their physician has moved to a new clinic site or the practice has relocated. Medical practices with Web sites can include a map of driving and parking directions on their site. And don't forget to include information about public transportation if needed.

Provide patients with a comprehensive practice brochure and/or Web site that describes your hours of operation, financial policies, locations, directions, services, etc. Patients who have easy access to this information won't need to call you for it.

Unnecessary calls

You may be receiving calls about issues that need not be addressed via the telephone. For example, if you round at an assisted living facility, your practice may receive dozens of calls each week from the facility's staff reporting minor injuries that are not emergencies but which must be reported. Evaluate your "frequent callers." Maybe there's an alternative form of communication you can use that would still fulfill your obligation to be informed but would not require a telephone call. Alternative forms of communication may include text paging, e-mail or fax. In this example, request the facility to fax or e-mail the non-emergency injury reports to you.

You can't get rid of all of these inbound calls – don't even think that you can just tell patients not to call – but you can reduce the number of calls somewhat with a little effort.

Reduce the rework

There are many steps you can take to reduce telephone demand and improve your telephone operations, but the most important step of all is to actually do the work and do it right the first time.

Incorporate the idea of a "virtual" exam room into each physician's schedule. Don't go anymore than four encounters before the physician addresses any outstanding messages, required documentation, and paperwork. Visit this virtual exam room several times an hour; don't leave all of this work until the end of the clinic or at the end of the day.

If you make the virtual exam room concept part of your day, you will reduce the amount of recall and rework time that is now likely part of your evening post-office hours ritual. It puts an end to patients calling your practice multiple times and your staff spending all that time recording, filing, batching, and organizing messages and paperwork.

For more information about the virtual exam room, see Chapter 7, "The Patient Encounter."

By attacking the work before it attacks you, you allow your staff the opportunity to better help your patients – and efficiently and effectively support the physician as he sees patients.

Summary of strategies to reduce telephone calls

✓ Establish office workflow so that transfers are unnecessary to avoid non-value-added time for you and your patients.

✓ Set a policy regarding the timing of callbacks to avoid unnecessary repeat calls from callers waiting for a response.

✓ Train your triage nurse to schedule appointments to avoid sending the caller back to the scheduler.

✓ Schedule follow-up appointments at checkout to reduce future appointment calls.

✓ Don't reschedule clinics to avoid the administrative work of rescheduling appointments.

✓ Conduct appointment reminders to reduce calls from forgetful patients about appointment date and time.

✓ Allow your schedulers to schedule so they aren't waiting instead of working.

✓ Manage the prescription process to reduce calls from patients and pharmacists.

✓ Promote your clinical team to patients so they can respond to their needs over the phone.

✓ Place a call to patients after a procedure or surgery to proactively handle questions.

✓ Take messages on labels to eliminate re-transcribing the information.

✓ Manage test results by effectively communicating to patients.

✓ Reduce clinical calls with proactive steps to educate patients.

✓ Schedule callbacks to reduce phone tag.

✓ Clarify statements to reduce bill calls.

✓ Anticipate general information requests to reduce calls about directions and policies.

✓ Handle information from frequent callers through other communication vehicles to reduce unnecessary calls.

✓ Reduce the rework.

Primary Care Associates makes staffing adjustments to control telephone demand

Problem: Primary Care Associates had an increasing volume of telephone calls coming in each day. Patients were complaining about long waits on hold when they called in to get test results. Schedulers felt swamped and frustrated as they tried to track down physicians and nurses to answer patients' medically related questions.

Observations: The practice had three full-time equivalent (FTE) schedulers who also handled any incoming telephone calls in which patients pressed "0" for operator. All three worked from 8:00 a.m. to 5:00 p.m.

To assess the volume of work they handled, the practice asked its telephone vendor to provide data regarding the number of calls handled per extension per day. The following graph was developed from the data.

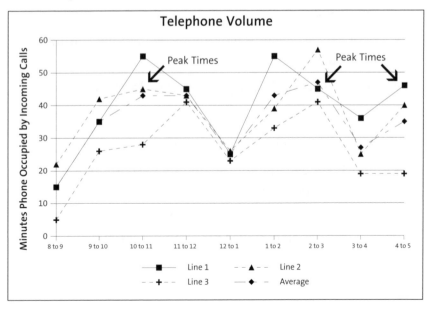

This graph shows call volume based on the amount of minutes occupied by incoming calls in each hourly block of time. As you can see, each operator had about 35 minutes of inbound calls per hour. However, the calls often came in clusters and many patients had to wait on hold. Simple graphing showed the practice that there was the potential for more flexible staffing without harming call coverage.

Analysis: Primary Care Associates had to do more than just add more lines and staff. Instead, each operational process was closely examined, not just the telephones. The practice discovered that the midlevel providers and physicians told their patients, "Give us a call to get your lab results" at the conclusion of the patients' visits. Patients, anxious about their results, began to call the following day. The providers did not realize that patients were calling so quickly, particularly because the majority of results were not in for 72 hours. Those calls had to be returned to tell patients that they would be called with results. Moreover, because no one had time to handle the callers who wanted to speak with a physician or nurse, those callers called back multiple times. The practice measured the callbacks from patients to be two calls per patient. Since patients were not receiving a return call in a timely manner, they would call the practice again. By observing its processes, the practice discovered that it was creating at least some of its own problem.

Solutions: Primary Care Associates reduced the number of schedulers/telephone operators from 3.0 full-time-equivalent (FTE) staff to 2.5 FTEs by staggering their work hours so that one operator came in early to open up the telephone lines at 7:45 a.m. and prepare other workstations for the day. The cost savings was used to increase nursing time by a couple hours per day to address return calls.

The practice installed telephones with voice mail at each nurses' station. Callers were initially "triaged" by the telephone operators to assure that emergencies were dealt with immediately and not sent to the nurses' voice mail. The lead nurse checked the voice-mail boxes at noon and 5:00 p.m. to assure that all messages had been cleared.

The practice established a new policy that all patient calls must be returned within two hours. This was enforced by tracking a sample of messages to ensure timeliness.

Providers made it a policy to tell patients that someone from the practice would call the patient with the test results in three days or as soon as results were in — and they adhered to this policy religiously.

Finally, Primary Care Associates implemented a policy of accepting prescription refills only from pharmacists (the practice's operators steered patients to call their pharmacy), and provided a dedicated fax line for pharmacists to transmit their requests to the practice.

Once patients realized that calls were being returned, lab tests reported, and prescriptions refilled in a timely manner, the inbound call volume decreased. By gathering data and considering its processes, the practice saved money, increased patient service, and decreased staff frustration.

Technology and telephones

If you still find yourself frustrated by the inability to handle your call volume, it's an opportune time to evaluate your telephone system and its components. Your telephone information system may need new features or you may need to learn more about its existing features. A multitude of functional options is now available to practices to employ; let's review a few of the most popular.

Telephone systems

Auto Attendant: System that answers and routes calls after prompting callers. For example, "Hello, you've reached Anytown Medical Associates. If you know your party's extension, please dial it now. Please dial 1 for appointments, 2 for the nurse, 3 for prescription refills, and 4 for billing and referrals. Dial 0 or hold for the operator."

Automatic Call Distributor (ACD) or **Uniform Call Distribution (UCD):** Software products that help telephone operators better manage incoming calls by distributing calls evenly to staff, pointing callers to specific functions (appointments, prescription refills, etc.), and placing callers on automatic hold – "in queue" – until a staff member is available to take the call. Can be used in place of or as a backup to your receptionist.

Call accounting: Software programs that capture, record, analyze and organize call data. The information is stored in a database that can be queried for operator productivity, call abandonment rate, and other analyses.

Call forwarding: Allows you to program the system to ring elsewhere if a station is busy or a call is not answered within a predetermined number of rings. Some systems permit external forwarding; some forward only within the system.

Call hunt: Bounces incoming calls automatically to the next available (not busy) line.

Call park: Allows you to place callers "in orbit," removing them from general telephone traffic in order to alert employees that a call is waiting.

Call transfer: Allows calls received from internal or external callers to be sent from one telephone to any other within the system.

Caller identification (ID): Allows you to identify the caller's registered name and number.

Capacity: The number of telephones, lines and software that a telephone system can handle. For example, a 24-port system can handle a combination of 24 lines and telephones.

Cellular Phone: A wireless telephone that can be transported with the user away from the docking station.

Central Processing Unit (CPU): The main cabinet that houses the system's intelligence and controls its activities.

Cordless Phone: A portable telephone that can fully integrate into your system, but which can be used from anywhere in your practice.

Custom Call Routing (CCR): Enables you to design custom routing points for callers – a big plus offered by some auto attendants. For example, a caller can leave a message in a mailbox and then be routed to specific locations within a practice.

Direct Inward Dialing (DID): Enables a caller to bypass the receptionist and go directly to the desired extension. DID trunks are assigned through the telephone company. Each trunk ordered has 24 associated telephones, each of which can be assigned to individual staff.

Integration: Combining telephone, fax and e-mail functions into a single system.

Interactive Voice Recognition (IVR): Software that prompts callers for information by asking them to use their telephone keypads or, in some systems, utter certain phrases in response to automated questions. IVR improves staff efficiency by routing callers to the appropriate staff based on information the caller provides.

Intercom: Enables you to ring another telephone within the system and talk internally without tying up an outside line.

Port: Point of connections in a system. Consider this the interface point at which programs are routed into the telephone system. A two-port voice-mail system enables two activities; a four-port voice-mail system allows four; an eight-port, eight. Ports are avenues that are open for travel once connected to a CPU.

Remote Notification: A pager or cell phone notifies the user that he or she has a voice-mail message.

T1: A digital transmission link with a capacity of 1.544 Mbps (1,544,000 bits of data per second). T1 normally can handle 24 simultaneous voice conversations or data links over two pairs of wires, each one digitized at 64 Kbps. This is accomplished by using special encoding and decoding equipment at each end of the transmission path to multiplex one circuit into 24 channels.

Traffic: The number of users on a call.

Trunk: A line or telephone number.

Voice mail

Is there a simple and cheap way to stop the flood of patient calls? Voice mail may be a solution. Many more practices are using voice mail. The reception tool of choice among corporate entities, voice mail allows busy staff to manage a fluctuating workload, thus increasing workflow efficiency and customer satisfaction.

Voice mail is a great way to improve the operation of your practice for certain functions. If designed and used properly, it can help your busy practice stay in business. If designed and used improperly, however, your loyal patients and referring physicians may quickly steer business away from you.

The use of voice mail can vary dramatically – from creating a single dedicated voice-mail box (for calls related to prescription refills, for instance) to giving staff personal voice-mail boxes. As a result, practices should be careful when deciding how to use voice mail.

If you are considering adding voice mail, first determine the needs and uses for it. Look at each area of your practice (billing, referrals, scheduling, staffing, etc.). Callers leaving a voice-mail message often expect a near-immediate response, especially if the question is urgent. Therefore, you may decide to give your billers voice-mail boxes, but not your nurses.

When choosing a voice-mail system, consider its reporting abilities. Sample activity reports should include the number of messages recorded, total length of messages, and average time before the message is deleted. These functions will help you monitor how your staff responds to messages from patients and referring physicians.

Also, consider how a voice-mail system indicates that a message is waiting. Is there a blinking light, an LCD (liquid crystal diode) display, or other visual cue to tell you that there's a new message in the system? Be sure that your system includes clear and succinct voice prompts that are user-friendly to internal staff members as well as to your patients and referring physicians.

Make sure that the system's port size and storage capacity are adequate for your needs. For example, how many messages can the voice-mail system hold? How long of a message can callers leave? What happens when the system is full?

And, training is as important as the system itself. Is the vendor's training comprehensive yet quick and simple? You don't want your staff spending days and days trying to learn the system; the transition should be seamless.

Of course, not everyone loves voice mail. Like an auto attendant, a complex system can easily frustrate callers, especially if they are given too many options but not offered the option to reach a live operator.

Choose an integrated voice-mail system, or one with interactive voice response (IVR) software that recognizes and adapts to usage patterns. Sophisticated IVR systems can route calls from one of your top referring physicians, for example, straight to your head nurse.

Callers and internal users should be able to locate their destinations easily in just one or two steps. Avoid a non-integrated system because it will not allow users to return to a menu after they leave their voice-mail message. As with a misused auto attendant, a non-integrated voice-mail system will bounce users from an extension where no one picks up, back to the greeting message, back to another unattended extension, back to the greeting, and so on – a potentially endless cycle, and one that could drive away patients and others.

In general, voice mail works best for the non-clinical functions of your practice, or at least those where there won't be an emergency that may lead to a bad outcome. These non-emergent uses for voice mail include billing, prescription refills, physician referrals, and office management. Although calls to these areas should be answered promptly, setting them aside for a short period should not lead to a risk-management problem.

WORDS OF WISDOM

Train, train, train

Training on your telephone system is just as important as training on your practice management system. Be sure to allocate enough time to orient and train new employees, as well as to educate everyone in your practice about upgrades and other changes.

Voice mail tips

- Use voice mail to back up staff who are on the telephone or otherwise unavailable.

- Always offer a "live" operator option so patients and others can get immediate assistance if needed.

- Check voice-mail boxes frequently to ensure fast response.

- Best used for billing, physician referral and prescription refill.

- Can become a risk management issue if used to triage clinical calls.

What to Avoid: Don't send callers to telephone jail

Great management tools like telephone auto attendants can turn into weapons if you are not careful. I called a practice recently and heard this after the greeting:

"Press 11 if you are a physician;
Press 9 if you want to speak to the billing office;
Press 16 for a referral;
Press 15 to schedule an appointment;
Press 7 to leave a message for the nurse;
Press 19 if you need test results;
Press 12 if you need a prescription refill;
If you know the extension of the person you wish to reach, you can press that at any time;
Press 10 to speak to an operator."

What impression does this give a patient? Does it say that your practice is a warm and caring place? That the staff are efficient? Or does it say that visiting your practice is going to be like standing in line all afternoon at the Department of Motor Vehicles?

Auto attendants

Another telephone feature to consider is an auto attendant. An auto attendant is a call processing system that answers calls and assists callers. Callers can route their calls by choosing options such as, "Press one for the triage nurse," "Press two for the billing department," "Press three for appointment scheduling," and so forth.

If unmanaged, auto attendants can backfire. Sometimes physicians react to the negative responses of what is often a small, but vocal, subset of patients by giving out their direct or "back line" telephone number. Before long, the "back line" becomes a main line. Thus, the auto attendant's cost savings are never realized as the practice struggles to manage multiple points of telephone entry.

Although patients expect to encounter auto attendants when calling credit-card companies, banks, airlines and government offices, they place higher demands on their physician's office. Patients interact with their physicians on a much more personal level than they do with their banks and are disappointed when it sounds like a computer is answering their physician's telephone.

Practices in rural areas and those with a large Medicare patient panel overwhelmingly reject this technology because their patients feel it is impersonal and difficult to use.

If you decide to use an auto attendant, deploy it with caution. Though potentially helpful for improving office workflow and saving money, the technology has some drawbacks for physician practices that must be carefully considered.

First, analyze the investment that you are about to make in the product. Solicit feedback from your entire practice, as it will affect everyone from the receptionist to the physicians. Ask: Will it save your practice money? Will it make your practice more efficient? Will it increase your response time to patients? If the answers to these questions are "no," then don't invest in an auto attendant.

Second, map your practice's workflow to ensure this new technology is used efficiently. Ensure that your callers will be responded to in a timely manner.

Third, carefully select the product and the vendor. Study the vendor's track record. Talk to several other practices that use the product. Negotiate a trial period to test the product, and don't skimp on service. Are all of these cautions really necessary? Yes! Your patients will never forgive you for losing their calls, and you'll put yourself into a risk-management situation.

Fourth, integrate the product. From day one, test it out yourself. Is it working? Spend a few minutes each day in your reception area asking patients for their opinions. Seek feedback from physicians and staff. Is it effective? Has it saved you money? Has it made your practice more efficient? Has it increased your response time to patients? Is your "return on investment" positive? Expect to use the system for at least six weeks before you see any impact on work flow.

If you have determined that the technology isn't right for your general number, consider its application for certain situations such as in the billing office, as a "back-up" for busy operators, for personal calls to employees, or for reaching a referral specialist.

Voice mail can be integrated with an auto attendant, allowing callers to leave a message at their chosen option if the requested staff member is unavailable. Essentially, the auto attendant takes the place of a receptionist routing calls to staff. If you choose this option, make sure it's user-friendly and allows your callers to choose "0" to reach the operator because some people prefer to speak to an operator or don't know which option they should choose.

Use auto attendants wisely

- List no more than five options so callers don't loose track and patience.

  Example:

  1. Schedule an appointment.
  2. Speak with a nurse.
  3. Discuss your bill.
  4. Refill a prescription.
  5. Speak with an operator.

- Number options "1" through "5" and list them in order;

- Always provide the option of a live operator and make sure there is a live operator;

- Before listing options, tell callers what to do if it's an emergency;

- Don't use an automated voice; ask a staff member to record;

- Deliver custom health messages to callers while on hold or being transferred;

- Use a system that allows you to see how long calls are waiting;

- Test your system weekly; and

- Offer non-English speaking callers an option.

Automatic call distributors

An automatic call distributor (ACD) – or a product with similar functionality called a uniform call distribution (UCD) – system can serve as a mechanism to distribute calls more effectively within the practice. The ACD software recognizes busy lines and places callers in waiting lines, distributing the calls to specific lines when they come free. Essentially, an ACD creates the opportunity for you to better route, handle, and categorize calls. Be sure to understand the storage capabilities of the system and what happens to overflow.

What to look for in an automatic call distributor

- Expandability

- Flexibility

- Wallboard support (displays incoming calls on a visible LED)

- Operators can attach callers to an auto attendant

- Callers can opt in or out of "queue"

- Silent monitoring

- Operators can log in and out

- Report generator

Telephony applications

Telecommunications software products (referred to collectively as "telephony") are now readily available for use in a medical practice. These software products integrate with your practice management system and/or your telephone to replicate or back up services that your staff currently provides. For example, you can purchase a product that integrates with your practice management system (the scheduling module, in particular) to use the schedule for the following day to remind patients of their appointments – the software finds the telephone numbers associated with each patient's name.

Try these computer telephony applications

- Appointment reminders and confirmation

- Lab results reporting

- Patient account balances

- Patient educational material requests

- Pre-recorded patient instructions and explanations

- Prescription refill requests

- Staff notification

- Patient satisfaction survey

Telephony helps MacArthur Surgical Clinic handle no-shows

One of the ongoing issues every medical office faces is the patient "no-show." At MacArthur Surgical Clinic, we asked ourselves, "How do we reduce the loss, increase our potential income and improve patient satisfaction?" Technology is certainly one way. With the installation of our new practice management software, local area network (LAN), new telephone system and upgraded computer equipment, we were well positioned to take advantage of telephony solutions.

One solution is a program called ReminderPro™. With a minimal amount of setup on our part, the program interfaces with the scheduling module of our practice management software and enables us to place a reminder call "computerly" to our patients two days prior to their appointment. The message, which can be customized, provides a mechanism for the patients to respond as to whether or not they will make their appointment.

Instead of finding out at 2:00 p.m. that our 2:00 p.m. patient is a no-show, we often now know what's what at 8:00 a.m. that morning or the day before. This allows us to either call the patient to reschedule or fill the slot with the numerous requests we get for same-day appointments.

No-shows are down, physicians at MacArthur are happy, the nurses are happy, and the patients are happy. Win-win all the way around.

Ken Hertz, Administrator, MacArthur Surgical Clinic, Alexandria, LA

Selecting or changing your telephone system

❑ Learn telephone system terms and procedures. Like health care, the telecommunications industry is full of acronyms and technical terminology. Knowing these terms will keep you on equal footing with your potential vendors.

❑ Learn the basic telephone equipment structure. Knowing the system's parts and features will help the process.

❑ Define your practice's needs. Review your existing system, as well as the features of the potential new system. Do you want voice mail, an auto attendant, automated call distribution, etc.?

❑ Involve your employees. Speaking with all of your staff to discuss specific needs, functions and ideas for functionality will help you choose the right system for your practice.

❑ Gather information and proposals from vendors. Select three to 10 vendors to submit a request for proposal (RFP) for your telephone system. The more specific you are, the more information you will garner from the proposals.

❑ Deal only with quality vendors. The telephone is your main communication portal to external customers (patients and referring physicians), as well as your internal network. Taking risks on an inexperienced vendor is foolish and may cause harm to your practice.

Don't let your telephone system compromise patient confidentiality

If your practice provides services that may be considered sensitive (psychiatry, obstetrics and infectious disease are a few that come to mind), consider blocking your practice's "caller identification (ID)" when calling patients. When you call patients to remind them of their appointment or report that their test results have arrived, your practice's name and number may appear on the recipient's caller ID display. This identification could compromise the patient's confidentiality if others in the household or business see it.

In addition to caller ID, consider answering your phones with the names of your physicians instead of the name of your specialty. For example, instead of using "Infectious Disease Consultants" in your telephone greeting, answer, "Drs. White and Smith." This will protect your patients' confidentiality in the case of "curious" family members or associates who redial your number from the caller ID.

While this concern may not be applicable to all types of medical practices or to all patients, keep in mind that some patients have higher demands for confidentiality. They may want to keep all of their medical affairs hidden from their family members as well as co-workers. If this is the case in your practice, be sure to ask your patients how best to handle communication from your practice. Put the request(s) in writing, with easy visibility in their chart. If you ask, you must be prepared to deliver – without any mistakes.

No matter what features or applications you consider, keep in mind the needs of your patient population. Pay special attention to the design of an automated system if large numbers of patients are not used to dealing with automated telephones or do not speak English. Remember to look at your current processes first to change telephone demand, followed by enhancing your operations changes by employing technology to help you – and your patients.

Staffing your telephones

Your performance improvement initiatives and a better telephone may help you better manage your phones, but they won't ever end the volume of phone calls – nor should they. Indeed, you'll always need staff to respond to calls. How many you need is the real question.

Using a system that has a messaging option, the average operator can respond to 300 to 500 phone calls per day. For example, the operator accepts the call, listens to the caller, records information about the caller's needs, and routes the message to the appropriate area of the practice. If the operator just routes calls, the productivity increases to 1,000 to 1,200 calls per day.

The average triage nurse can respond to 65 to 80 calls per day. But, before you add to your triage nurse staff, utilize the Incoming Clinical Calls Log on page 58 to evaluate where calls could be avoided altogether by improving patient education while patients are in the office. Further, scrutinize the calls regarding issues that may have been better handled in the office face-to-face with a clinician. As patients seek more "telephone medicine" and only a handful of insurance companies reimburse for it, your practice is being stuck with the overhead. If the patient would be better off coming in, then go ahead and make the appointment.

Estimate your staffing needs based on how you have configured your telephone operations and the benchmarks listed above. Don't ever take benchmarks at pure face value – if an operator must walk from the desk to deliver every message to the nurses' station, for example, then adjust the benchmark accordingly.

A warning about staffing your phones: telephone staffs, like all of us, have a tendency to pace their work to match the demands of the moment. For example, a busy practice looked for ways to reduce staff. During its telephone analysis, the practice realized that the volume of incoming telephone calls was much greater on Mondays, then decreased as the week went on. However, on Fridays, even though the call volume was lower, the operators' time on the telephone was higher per call. Staff complained that they needed more help. But when the practice analyzed the situation, the results were surprising. As the phones rung less, the staff talked longer. The operators spent 25 percent more time per call on Fridays because they expanded their efforts to match the demands of the moment. Since there were more moments (and fewer calls), there was more talking.

Staffing Compared to Volume

Day of Week	Operator Time (Hrs)	Telephone Volume*	Seconds per Call
Monday	19.15	1200	57.5
Tuesday	11.29	700	58.1
Wednesday	8.54	650	47.3
Thursday	7.99	620	46.4
Friday	11.68	589	71.4

Not displayed in the graph.

Length of Operator Calls

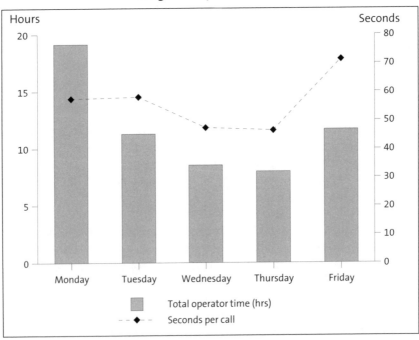

This is a natural phenomenon, but it's often hidden. Even the manager thought that the practice needed another operator. You can't do much to prevent the expansion-of-effort phenomenon, but don't let it lead you to increase overhead unnecessarily. In this example, the practice simply hired another operator to work on Mondays, thus saving more than 80 percent of the cost of a full-time employee because the part-time worker did not receive benefits.

A final word on telephone management

Managing telephone demand is not a one-time solution. It's continuous. Evaluate technology and staff costs each year. Better communication in the office and with patients will cut the volume of unnecessary telephone calls, reduce your overhead and staffing costs, and increase patient satisfaction. Focus your efforts on managing the demand and you will reap rewards for your practice and your patients.

ADVANCED CONCEPT

HIPAA and your telephone

HIPAA is the acronym for the Health Insurance Portability and Accountability Act, a law that was designed – among other things – to develop standards to protect the security and privacy of patient health information.

HIPAA requires that a "reasonable" effort be made to protect a patient's privacy. HIPAA does not specifically address the role of telephones in a physician's office but it does give guidelines that can be applied to the situation.

General: Base your telephone policies on sound business practices, common sense, and the use and disclosure of the minimum protected health information required to perform the specific task.

Position of operators: You need not build a soundproof room in your practice for your telephone operators, but move them from a location where other patients may overhear private information. This should apply to your triage nurses as well.

Reminder calls: Include a statement in your Notice of Privacy Practices that you place reminder calls, or develop a patient consent form for reminder calls in your new patient registration materials. You have to respect your patients' wishes, so if you encourage exceptions about the method of notification, be sure to have the ability to handle them without any mistakes. If a patient declines to have a reminder altogether, have a procedure in place to respect this request.

Develop a written policy for information to leave on patients' voice-mail or answering machines. The HIPAA rules merely say you need to limit information to the minimum necessary; they don't specify what should be included or excluded. Industry practice has been to limit the information to patient's name, date, time and physician's last name. An example is: "This message is for Jane Doe. You have an appointment with Dr. Jones on Tuesday at 2:00 p.m." Do not include the specialty of your practice or the nature of the appointment.

Unless there are extenuating circumstances, do not be overly concerned about a relative getting the message instead of or as well as your patient. HIPAA encourages physicians to be in communication with their patients and does allow physicians to communicate minimum necessary information to family members or other caregivers as they see fit to benefit the patient.

If your reminders are communicated through the mail, use these same guidelines about minimal information.

E-mail: You can send e-mail to patients, pharmacies, referring physicians and others, but it should be encrypted. HIPAA's Privacy Rule requires you to create "reasonable safeguards" to protect health information, and encryption seems a fairly minimal step. HIPAA's Security Rule, with which practices must comply by 2005, may enforce stricter standards, but, as of the date of this book's publication, interpretation of that rule remains rather vague. Nonetheless, be sure to confer with an attorney familiar with the Security Rule before investing in this area for the long term. To transmit and receive encrypted e-mail, both users will need to use the same encryption software and have a personal digital identification number. Microsoft Outlook has a simple encryption tool, and there is a medley of encryption software companies and web-based services, as well as secure web servers through which to transmit secure e-mail.

Test results: Again, HIPAA doesn't specifically address test results, but sound business judgment would mean that you do not leave test results on a patient's voicemail, answering machine or e-mail account without his permission.

Revisit these important issues on a quarterly basis to make sure that your telephone operations keep up with federal and state regulations.

Chapter 4

SCHEDULING

Key Chapter Lessons

> Evaluate your scheduling process

> Learn the common scheduling methodologies

> Identify scheduling bottlenecks to make improvements

> Evaluate same–day appointment requests

> Use advanced access to make your day run smoother

> Integrate staff resources with your appointment schedule

> Understand scheduling fluctuations and how to measure them

> Recognize the root cause of "no-shows" and how to reduce them

> Examine "bumped" appointments and their financial effect

> Learn to conduct the surgery scheduling process more effectively

> Identify the steps to facilitate appointment recalls and appointment reminders

Advanced Concepts

> Preappointment screening

> Physician supply and patient demand

> Group visits

> Express clinics

Scheduling: the key to better patient flow

Once you successfully field a call from a patient, you must find a place for that patient in the schedule.

Scheduling is a crucial step in the patient flow process. Scheduling impacts the entire patient flow process, getting it off to a smooth start, a rocky beginning or somewhere in between.

Good scheduling demands good planning, good data, good information systems and, above all, good staff; that is, workers who are trained, committed and empowered to provide top-notch customer service.

Scheduling practices impact administrative and clinical performance

Higher patient volume generally leads to more practice revenue before fixed and variable expenses are subtracted. Ah, those fixed expenses. They include the great number of non-clinical tasks that go along with patient volume. Copayments must be collected, telephones must be answered, forms must be filled out and numerous scheduling tasks must be handled. However, the fixed costs remain in place whether the physician sees 30 patients a day or 10 patients, or takes the day off.

While patient revenue and variable costs like supplies do fluctuate along with patient volume, fixed costs remain fixed. Or do they? Actually, fixed costs can increase, but usually because of poor planning, not because there are more patients visiting the practice. Sloppy scheduling can cause administrative staff to work harder and do less.

When it comes to scheduling and its impact, here's a simple formula to remember:

Bad scheduling practices = Higher fixed costs (staff time) = Reduced patient volume = Less revenue = More time that physicians must spend to produce enough revenue after expenses to sustain the practice

See Chapter 10, "Fundamental Financials," for more information regarding fixed and variable costs.

Do you need to rethink your scheduling process?

❑ How many staff members must patients speak to when trying to schedule appointments?

❑ How long must patients wait on hold when they call to schedule an appointment?

❑ How many times are patients trying to schedule appointments put on hold and transferred to other staff?

❑ Do schedulers have to ask physicians or others for permission before scheduling patients?

❑ Do "no-shows" continually play havoc with the practice's daily schedule?

❑ Do physicians run on time some days but get completely behind on other days for no apparent reason?

❑ Do you have trouble making room for same-day appointments?

Poor scheduling can cost your practice money: fewer patients are seen and the physician's valuable time is wasted.

Scheduling snafus frustrate staff, too. A muddled scheduling process puts them directly in the line of fire from angry patients. Sometimes, staff responsible for scheduling get so fed up with the logjams that they will try to help patients by suggesting other physicians in the community who can fit them in. Don't blame the staff when it might be the scheduling system or the process itself that's at fault.

Medical practices use three general methods of scheduling: single interval, multiple interval and block, or wave, intervals. In brief, these methods operate as follows:

Single intervals: Each visit receives the same amount of time on the scheduling calendar, regardless of the type of visit (new or established) or chief complaint (health check or asthma). An example is scheduling all appointments on the quarter hour.

Multiple intervals: The intervals between appointments depend on the type of visit or the patient's chief complaint(s). For example, an acute care visit with a single complaint would receive 15 minutes on the scheduling calendar while a new patient visit would be given 30 minutes.

Block (wave) intervals: There is a single block of time for multiple appointments regardless of the type of visit or the patient's chief complaint. For example, all 12 morning appointments are asked to present at 9:00 a.m. and are seen in some predetermined order until the end of that morning's clinic.

Most practices use the second methodology – multiple intervals – because it allows them to take into account the approximate amount of time a patient may need while maintaining awareness of the patient's waiting time.

Communicating to your new patient

When a patient calls for an appointment, the initial telephone call is your chance to describe any attributes or policies regarding your practice that you wish to convey prior to the patient showing up at your front office.

Consider the following:

✓ Thank the patient for choosing your practice;

✓ Ask the patient from where or whom he was referred;

✓ Indicate the length of time a patient can expect to be at your office for the appointment;

✔ Mention the contingency plan for contacting the patient if the physician must tend to an emergency (and make sure you get the patient's contact information);

✔ Ask the patient how he or she would like to be addressed at your practice;

✔ Remind the patient of any dietary or other preparations for the visit;

✔ Describe the practice's policy regarding patient payments at the time of service; and

✔ Tell him that you look forward to him coming next week. You can reduce the frustrations felt by many patients by simply keeping them informed about the encounter and always being courteous.

Simpler scheduling

Don't take multiple intervals to an extreme, however. Many practices have dozens – if not hundreds – of appointment types. Staff spends precious minutes trying to determine if the patient fits into a "return-acute long" or a "return-acute medium." One practice I visited had appointment slots for "short," "short-short," "short-short-short," "long," "long-long" and "long-long-long" appointments. Of course, when the patient arrives she rarely fits neatly into one of these categories anyway.

Our complicated system of appointment types creates extra overhead – with little to no value to the practice. What does the patient care if she is a "long" or a "long-long-long?" She doesn't – she just wants to be seen. So, why spend hours developing, maintaining and training staff on appointment types that rarely accomplish the goal of predicting the length of the appointment? It makes no sense.

Release your practice from the burden of a complicated scheduling template. Simplify the scheduling model. Limit appointment types to as few as possible. Many physicians are moving to scheduling office appointments in three basic categories: short (usually established patients), long (usually new patients and complex established patients) and procedures. There may be exceptions to this simplification, but don't let the exceptions take over the process.

If you adopt a simple schedule, you'll see more patients, reduce your staffing costs and have less frustrated staff.

Too many appointment types

I visited a practice that had 1,100 different appointment categories. The schedulers had thick notebooks with instructions about each appointment type that they had to consult with every time a patient called. Not only were the schedulers' salaries low but they also had to bear the brunt of physicians' and patients' frustrations when the scheduling process, which no one could master, inevitably broke down. It was no wonder that their scheduling staff turnover was high.

Make sure that you haven't given your schedulers an impossible job.

Treat your schedulers well

It may be time to take a hard look at your schedulers' working conditions. Do they:

✓ Work in a crowded, unpleasant space?

✓ Have to get up every five minutes and ask physicians for permission to make appointments?

✓ Struggle with an inefficient scheduling system or outdated software?

✓ Receive disrespectful treatment from physicians and staff?

✓ Lack work incentives – not even nonmonetary rewards like simply saying "thank you" once in a while?

If you answered yes to any of these questions, then get to work to improve your most valuable scheduling resource: your schedulers. Give them appropriate pay, a respectful work environment and the tools they need to do their jobs. They'll stick around longer – and keep your practice on track.

Modified wave

Some practices modify the multiple interval methodology, often by using a modified wave approach.

A long or more complicated patient visit is scheduled at the same time as a visit of shorter duration. This double booking can allow the physician to begin serving the short visit while her clinical assistant prepares the longer visit. For example, scheduling a well-woman visit and a sore throat patient to both begin at 9:00 a.m. allows the patient getting the well-woman check-up time to undress, be weighed and do other intake activities under the direction of the physician's clinical assistant. Meanwhile, the physician handles the acute-visit patient whose visit is shorter.

Access

We call them patients but they are hardly patient anymore. Service providers in every industry are struggling to reduce wait times.

Your average time to next available appointment for new patients is especially critical; your practice's growth depends how well you accommodate new patients.

Here's an example. Your practice's newest internist saw 25 patients a day during her first two years with your group. By her fifth year of practice you notice that she is producing less revenue, even though she still sees 25 patients a day. What happened? Most of her patients during those early years were new patients. Their visits generated more revenue than established patients with similar medical complaints.

Now, most of her patients are established patients, many of whom have chronic conditions. Solution? Better management of this physician's patient access can allow her to see some new patients.

The appropriate time to the next available appointment varies by specialty. For a trauma surgeon, it may be the next hour; for an endocrinologist, it may not be for two weeks.

Patients who cannot get prompt access can get sicker or become well on their own. The former situation is a risk management issue and the latter scenario boosts your no-show rate. Alternatively, patients frustrated by long time-to-next-appointment waits may go to one of your competitors or show up at the emergency room.

Let your patients' needs determine the ideal time to your next open appointment slot. Set a goal and make it a point to measure your practice against this benchmark every month. If you fail to meet your benchmark, you have two options: decrease demand or increase capacity.

Access performance dashboard

☐ **Time to Next Available New Patient Appointment**
(Number of days to next available appointment slot that can accommodate a new patient)

☐ **Time to Next Available Established Patient Appointment**
(Number of days to next available appointment slot that can accommodate an established patient)

☐ **Appointment No-Show Rate**
(Percent of appointments that patients do not keep; that is, the appointment is scheduled but the patient doesn't show up)

☐ **Appointment "Bump" Rate**
(Percent of appointments that the physician cancels in which patients must be "bumped")

❑ **New Patient Appointments as a Percent of Total Appointment.**
(Percent of new patient appointment slots as a percent of total appointment slots)

❑ **Cancellation Conversion Rate**
(Percent of cancelled appointments that are converted to an appointment in which another patient is seen – often, through a waiting list or accommodating a patient who calls in the meantime)

Health plans measure access

The notion of access is not just a concern on the part of your patients; health plans have begun to measure access to your medical practice – on the telephone and for an appointment. Here's a survey for your patients:

1. When you leave your physician a telephone message, how long does it usually take to receive a return call?

2. When you are ill (e.g., back pain, headache) and you call to see your physician, how soon is the appointment scheduled from the time you call?

3. When the office is closed and you need to reach your physician or the covering physician, how long does it take for the physician to return your call?

4. Please rate the timeliness of your ability to contact your physician during office hours. How long does it take for the physician to see you after you arrive for your visit?

Source: Fallon Community Health Plan, Worcester, MA

Same-day appointments

We'd like to give patients the swift service that our digital, instant access economy is conditioning them to expect. That's not always practical, but many medical practices are trying to handle walk-ins and same-day appointments more successfully to meet patients' demands for swifter access.

Many practices hold open a portion of each day's time slots until the day before or until the same day to accommodate last-minute requests for appointments.

The slots may be kept open in each physician's schedule and accommodated by a nurse practitioner or physician assistant, or handled by a physician who is designated as the "doctor of the day."

Although it's easier to assign one physician as the acute caregiver, it should be noted that it's generally not as efficient. The inefficiency stems from the fact that the physicians are seeing someone else's patients and having to read someone else's notes, lab results, treatment plans and so forth. Further, depending on the specialty, at the end of the "doctor-of-the-day" encounter, the patient is often told to schedule an appointment with his regular physician because only the acute need was addressed. Many practices find that the "doctor-of-the-day" model simply delays when the patient sees his own physician; it doesn't actually satisfy the patient's demands.

No matter how you accommodate your appointment requests from patients with acute needs, you need to consider the question: How many appointment slots should I hold open each day to handle acute appointment requests?

Conducting an analysis of appointment requests and fulfillment will help you to determine how many appointment slots your practice needs to hold open. The analysis works for both the doctor-of-the-day model and the open access to all physicians model.

Use your practice's own data. How many requests for same-day appointments do you really have? How many of these requests does your practice fulfill? Track the number of each using this appointment request and fulfillment analysis tracking form for at least a month.

Appointment Request and Fulfillment Analysis Tracking Form

Name: _____

Week: _____

	Morning					
	New Patient			Established Patient		
	Requests?	Fulfilled?	Percent	Requests?	Fulfilled?	Percent
Monday						
Tuesday						
Wednesday						
Thursday						
Friday						

	Afternoon					
	New Patient			Established Patient		
	Requests?	Fulfilled?	Percent	Requests?	Fulfilled?	Percent
Monday						
Tuesday						
Wednesday						
Thursday						
Friday						

It may also help to track the peak days of the week and month, as there is often variability among these. For example, practices often see an increased demand for acute visits on Mondays. Track requests by morning and afternoon, as they may vary as well.

You may also notice seasonal trends that impact scheduling. Pediatricians, family physicians, internists, allergists and other specialists may need to seasonally adjust the number of walk-in and same-day slots to account for flu and allergy seasons and back-to-school physicals.

Take the data that you have gathered and use the 80-percent rule of thumb to dictate the number of slots to be held open. If the practice averages five same-day appointments a day, then hold four slots open at the very end of the day. Cancellations and no-shows can often create the additional slot that you will need. If your practice never has cancellations or no-shows, ignore the 80 percent and simply hold open exactly the number of slots you've determined in your analysis of demand.

Also, look at how many same-day appointments you are contractually obligated to schedule. Some insurance companies may stipulate that their patients must be seen within 24 hours of request. Calculate the percentage of your practice's patients that fall under such rules. If it is 10 percent of the practice's patients, and each physician sees 30 patients on a normal day, then you may need to hold two or three slots open per physician. Also take into account the demographics, such as average age, of the insurance companies' patient population that may impact utilization.

Advanced access

If you are frustrated by calculating the exact number of slots to hold open or if you find yourself trying to protect the last remaining slot from patients who don't "deserve" it, then you'll want to consider advanced access.

 ...you are just protecting the schedule when you tell patients:

— "Let me transfer you to the nurse. She can help you with your [medical] problem over the phone."

— "Sounds like you need to come in, but let me check with the doctor."

— "Just how sick are you? How red is the blood? Is it really red, or is it brown? If it's brown, then it's old and we can see you tomorrow."

— "We can't see you, but you need to be seen, so go to the emergency room." [Then, after seeing your patient, the ER physician declares, "call your regular physician to make an appointment to see him about this issue!"]

Most often, you spend more energy and time protecting your schedule than any value that protection adds. Do you think that an insurance company or a patient pays for this protection? Think again!

Advanced access is leaving your entire appointment schedule – except previously scheduled new patient and follow-up visits – open to patients who call with acute needs and want to be seen in short order. The patient sees her own physician – or, at least, her own care team, not a designated "doctor of the day." Advanced access can make your practice more accessible to patients, get new patients in faster, reduce no-show rates and make the entire scheduling process run smoother.

Although it seems quite daunting for practices that routinely book appointment weeks – even months – in advance, it's business as usual for many specialties. Take an oncology practice, for example – when a referring physician calls the oncologist with news that one of his patients has a large mass in her breast, does the scheduler at the oncology practice respond, "It'll be six weeks before she can get into see us!" If they did, they'd be out of business – and may even have some malpractice cases on their hands. The point is that advanced access is a fancy term, but it simply means being able to accommodate your patients when they – or their referring physicians – desire.

Advanced access, however, is more than just a scheduling methodology. It's a change of attitude, work style and even culture. Practices with backlogs often carry the same backlog over time – if measured on January 1st, for example, the backlog of appointments is six weeks, and measured again on July 1st, it's still six weeks. If the backlog is consistent, then the laws of supply and demand would empower us to say, why can't it be *zero weeks*, thus eliminating the backlog altogether?

Advanced Access: Supply and Demand in Equilibrium

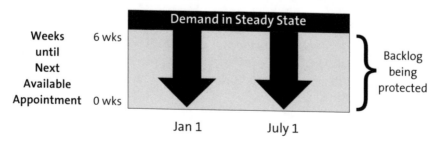

When a practice matures, the backlog often becomes a part of the practice and is not challenged. When it becomes part of the practice, here's what happens:

- Staff spend more time attempting to determine whether patients who call in with acute needs "deserve" an appointment.
- Staff spends more time giving medical advice over the telephone.
- Staff doesn't have as much time to assist the physician.

These activities are not reimbursed by our current reimbursement system; that is, neither insurance companies nor patients pay you for maintaining your backlog.

Of course, you welcomed those acute appointment calls when you first opened your practice, but many practices shift focus as the practice matures. And that shift significantly hurts access, efficiency and profitability.

If you've moved from welcoming patients to protecting physicians from patients' demands, advanced access may be the solution for you.

Advanced access principles

The four principles of advanced-access scheduling are:

1. The continuity of the patient/physician relationship is fundamental to fulfilling the patient's needs.

2. Processing work on a real-time basis is critical to cost-effectiveness and efficiency.

3. Success in creating timely access requires a balance between physician supply and patient demand.

4. When physician supply and patient demand are in equilibrium, the practice can accommodate all of today's appointment requests today.

The **continuity of the patient/physician relationship** is fundamental to fulfilling patients' needs. Patients want to see "their" physician for acute visits but often are scheduled to see a covering physician. Many patients end up seeing their chosen physician a minority of the time. When patients are able see their own physicians, their demand for additional appointments often decreases. Moreover, patient satisfaction increases significantly.

Processing work on a real-time basis is critical to be cost effective and efficient. Delays create unnecessary expenses. Here's a way many practices cause unnecessary delays: patients' telephone messages are taken by an operator, evaluated by a medical assistant, reviewed by a physician and return calls are made by a nurse. This messaging process may take an hour or an entire day to complete.

Because it is difficult for patients to get timely access to care, or even get their telephone calls returned in a timely manner, many try alternative routes to get the care they feel they need. When that happens, the practice has the additional burden of managing the alternative routes patients use to get care. As a result, practice resources, including a great deal of administrative and clinical staff time, are spent on fulfilling patients' interim needs and deflecting their demand.

It is usually more efficient to schedule appointments when patients call rather than routing their requests through so many channels. Hand-offs and forms reduce the time that staff can productively spend in patient care (and billable activities). It is more efficient to spend time on patient visits instead of finding ways to keep them out of the practice.

Success in creating timely access is dependent on a **balance between physician supply and patient demand.** In order to meet patients' demands, there must be a reasonable supply of physicians. For example, a family practitioner cannot possibly meet the appointment demands of 20,000 patients seeking care but can certainly meet the demands of 2,000. A practice — of any specialty — must supply enough care to meet the demands of the population of patients that it serves.

If the wait time is growing, then supply and demand are out of balance. When average wait times lengthen, a practice should consider improving efficiency in the office, do better time management or recruit an additional physician.

When physician supply and patient demand are in equilibrium, the **practice can accommodate today's appointment requests today.** Practices that consistently have long waiting times to the next available appointment have the opportunity to match supply and demand. When demand exceeds supply, the time to the next available appointment will increase over time. However, many practices have consistent access gaps. That is, it took 45 days to see a new patient last March and 45 days this March. If the time is the same (that is, demand is not growing faster than the supply of appointments), there is no reason why the time to the next available appointment can't – and shouldn't – be zero days.

For more information on determining when demand outstrips supply, see the Advanced Concept on measuring supply and demand at the end of this chapter.

Backlogs develop over time and, in a way, provide comfort to many physicians because they perceive long wait times as indications of their popularity. Statistically, backlogs should be unnecessary if wait times are stable.

Advanced access for specialists

If your specialty practice relies on getting referrals and needs authorizations before providing services, you may have to modify the concept of advanced access. Referral-dependent practices often need two or three days to get insurance companies' authorizations for referred patients. If so, consider those two to three days the equivalent of zero days when measuring the time to the next available appointment.

Here are the steps to fully integrate advanced access scheduling into your practice:

Educate stakeholders. Patients, physicians and staff must believe in advanced access. Patients will be surprised to learn that they can be seen the same day that they call for an appointment. Physicians will be anxious about having an open schedule when they walk in every morning. Staff may instinctively try to deflect demand for appointments to other days, thinking that this helps keep physicians' schedules open.

Work through the backlog. Your practice must first eliminate its backlog of patients waiting for appointments. If your time to next-available appointment is five weeks, it will take your practice at least five weeks, but possibly six weeks, to accomplish this objective.

Words of wisdom about scheduling backlogs

Here are some tips to work through your scheduling backlog:

- Contact patients whose appointments are several weeks away, and open up an evening or two a week or a Saturday or two to accommodate them sooner.

- Pull work into the day – if you see a patient who has a physical scheduled in two weeks, handle it today.

- Evaluate the scheduled follow-up appointments to find any patients whom you could call and touch base with over the telephone instead seeing in the office.

- Look at what other members of the team could do. Could a physician assistant see some patients? Can a nurse screen patients over the phone before their visits?

- Consider group visits – you can see more patients and achieve higher satisfaction in less time. (See the Advanced Concept section at the end of this chapter for more information on group visits.)

Whittling down your backlog takes physician and staff dedication, but it can be done.

Develop an effective process for record retrieval. Because many patients will be scheduled on a same-day basis, your records staff must be able to fulfill requests rapidly. An electronic medical record makes this step easy.

Prepare for variability. Physicians and staff may have to stay late once in a while.

Plan for contingencies. What happens if patient demand exceeds physician capacity on some days? Do you have back-up plan? Ask midlevel providers to serve as back up to physicians when demand exceeds the availability of appointments. If your practice does not employ midlevel providers, can a physician agree to take on the rare day when all of the physicians are overloaded? If you predict demand with accuracy, you won't need to access your contingency plan very often, but it's still good to have one.

Schedule patients with their chosen physicians. The continuity of the patient-physician relationship is essential to advanced access scheduling. Overloads are infrequent if you plan for advanced access scheduling. Ask part-time physicians to team up to function as a full-time physician. To accomplish this, tell patients that the part-time physicians are now a team.

Empower staff to meet patient needs. For example, manage telephone messages on a real-time basis, instead of just handing callers off to other staff. The more handoffs, the greater the chances of miscommunication.

Speed internal communications. Figure out how to improve communication between the front desk and the back office. Invest in better intercoms, more computer terminals, and intranet and telephonic technology as needed. Maybe you can rearrange space to put clerical and clinical staff in closer physical proximity.

Eliminate appointment distinctions (i.e., routine versus urgent). Multitudinous appointment types become irrelevant under advanced access, although you should continue to distinguish new patients from established patients for administrative and clinical purposes.

Plan for the visit. At the time an appointment is scheduled, ask patients if there is anything that they need taken care of during the appointment. Seek accurate information at the point of appointment scheduling to be prepared for the visit (e.g., liquid nitrogen to remove a skin wart) by stating, "Ms. Jones, Dr. Smith wants to be prepared for your visit tomorrow; can you tell me what you are coming in for?" Look in the chart for upcoming immunizations, well-woman checks and so forth. Meet with your staff at the beginning of each clinic session to anticipate patients' needs. Pull that work into today.

Complete the visit. Don't deflect work until later in the day. Dictate the note, finalize the paperwork, send the referral, or transmit the prescription to the pharmacy at the time the request or need arises. Consider the length of your appointments. Many practices find that they need to increase the spacing of appointments (for example, from every 15 minutes to every 20 minutes) if paperwork is included. In doing this, remember that real-time work is more efficient than batching work. You may find that you can reduce the two hours spent doing paperwork each day by incorporating portions of that time into each patient's visit. It can reduce the length of your workday.

Don't cluster follow-up visits. Schedule patients' follow-up visits as needed but don't always put them on Mondays, for example. If Mondays are busy days, then schedule follow-up visits on other weekdays.

Let patient demand manage physician supply, not the other way around. If 1,000 new patients sign up with your practice, then seek temporary help immediately while you recruit a permanent physician to meet the increased demand. Schedule vacations in a similar fashion. The majority of your physicians should not go on vacation during the weeks or months that patient demand normally peaks for your specialty (e.g., flu season). You'll know there is an imbalance between your physicians' capacity and your patients' service demands when you see time-to-next-available-appointment numbers increasing (that's why you track how long it is to the next-available appointment).

Spread the word. Greet patients with information about your new advanced access scheduling policy so they won't be surprised when they can be seen quickly.

Advanced Access in a Residency Clinic

Residency clinics may find it impossible to embrace advanced access because the notion of a physician/patient relationship cannot exist with faculty members who spend a few half-days in the clinic each week and residents who change rotations every few weeks. If you held on to the principles of advanced access, any full-time clinical faculty that you do have would find their schedules booked up – and out – and the residents left with an empty schedule.

Despite these obstacles, advanced access can still work, with one caveat: Change the principle of a "physician/patient" relationship to a "care team/patient" relationship.

Establish a care team with several faculty members and residents – at least one provider in the care team should be there five days a week. Then, assign a nurse(s) to each care team. Then, apply the principles of advanced access to the care team. Patients' acute requests should be scheduled with this care team, and the nurse(s) can provide the day-to-day continuity for the team.

Words of wisdom about follow-ups

Never schedule follow-ups on Mondays (unless the patient specifically requests it). Advanced access will require more slots to be available on Monday. Plan for it by avoiding follow-ups on Mondays.

Words of wisdom about why advanced access works

- Patients love it. They get to be seen when they want.

- Physicians love it. They get to see their own patients, which is more professionally rewarding.

- Practices love it. They are more efficient; instead of spending time deflecting demand, they use the same amount of resources to see more patients faster it.

- Risk managers love it. Fewer clinical issues fall through the cracks because patients are seen more promptly.

- Physician owners and managers love it. Gross charges, collections and income are higher.

Among the many benefits of advanced access are that it:

- Increases patient satisfaction;

- Enhances physician efficiency;

- Allows you to provide swifter service, which our instant-access economy is conditioning patients to expect;

- Fulfills your patients' needs today;

- Decreases your appointment no-show rate;

- Improves your performance ratings by insurance companies that set access standards;

- Enhances your coordination of care because patients see their own physicians;

- Enhances your market position as access attracts new patients who could not get timely appointments with your competitors;

- Improves your relationships with referring physicians;

- Reduces resources spent to create barriers to access your practice;

- Reduces your malpractice risk because you aren't deflecting your patients' problems;

- Ensures your compliance with insurance contracts that demand 24-hour access for their beneficiaries;

- Reduces the time spent explaining poor access;

- Increases the level of work per visit (i.e., more RVUs); and

- Improves physician satisfaction because physicians see their own patients.

Advanced access boosts RVUs

Advanced access helps physicians increase their production of relative value units (RVUs) because:

- More work is done during each visit;

- No-show rates decrease dramatically;

- More patients are seen – both new and established – because the practice is more efficient (e.g., nurses are nurses instead of deciding whether to schedule an appointment); and

- More surgeries and procedures are performed because there are more new patients, therefore, gross charges, collections and income are higher.

Advanced access requires flexibility and preparation. Rigid scheduling templates aren't allowed and appointments scheduled today cannot become a crisis. Further, it will fail if your practice never gets through its appointment backlog.

Advanced access offers a useful solution to a problem that is growing worse throughout our nation's health care system.

Implementation of advanced access is not effortless, but remaining focused on your patients' needs will make the transition easier.

If implemented and managed properly, advanced access scheduling will boost your practice's operational performance, reduce risk, increase profitability and keep patients coming back.

Words of wisdom about primary care panels and advanced access

For primary care practices, between 0.75 and 1 percent of your patients will seek care each day. If offered a same-day appointment, 75 percent of adults and 80 percent of children would accept it.

For a panel of 2,500 active patients, this means that 20 to 25 patients will seek care each day, whether on their own initiative or because you've scheduled a follow-up visit for them. Of course, this can fluctuate based on the severity of your patient panel, your follow-up protocols and seasonal issues (flu season, school physicals, etc.).

Source: Mary Murray, MD, Murray, Tantau and Associates

Monitoring advanced access

Monitor your time to next available appointment closely. If you find demand exceeding supply, check the following areas:

Follow up visit protocols. Are physicians bringing patients back in out of habit? Can the nurse check on patients by telephone? Can the physicians do that work today instead of 3 weeks from now? If so, they can likely bill for a higher-level visit *and* allow that future appointment slot to be taken by a new patient.

Operational efficiency. Make sure that you're as efficient as possible. Do you have supportive staff and facilities? Is everyone doing the right work the right way?

Midlevel provider and physician capacity. If the practice has maxed out its efficiency, maybe it's time to add another provider. (See the Advanced Concept on measuring supply and demand at the end of this chapter for more information on determining when it's time to recruit another provider.)

Insurance companies. Before you add another provider, look at the profile of your patients' insurance companies. Although not recommended in most cases, your practice could close to new patients. Alternately, target which part of the panel to close by performing a cost/benefit analysis of each insurance company when its contract comes up for renewal. Consider not renewing one or more of the contracts with insurance companies that reimburse your practice below cost or below your market's average.

If advanced access is too radical for your practice, review the following tips designed to make scheduling easier – and your practice more productive.

Fast-track clinic helps handle same-day appointments

CASE STUDIES

Noticing an increase in same-day appointment requests during the winter months, Northeast Pediatric Partners initiated a fast-track clinic. The daily session, which they called "KidsExpress," was held each morning from 7:00 to 9:00 a.m., and featured 15-minute appointment slots. One physician and one midlevel provider handled each morning's session. The arrangement allowed parents to bring their children in for urgent problems. The rotating assignments allowed the physicians and midlevel providers to work more flexible schedules. In addition, the physicians on night call received fewer calls from parents because they knew they could bring their child in the next morning. By grouping the visits (and interspersing school physicals and new patient appointments), the providers found themselves more productive, and with much happier parents. (See the Advanced Concept, "Express Clinics," at the end of this chapter for more information.)

Delegate scheduling duties DOWN...

One way to make the scheduling process run faster and smoother is to reduce the number of times a patient is transferred or put on hold. Allow the staff members who already handle telephone duties to also schedule appointments. Placing the necessary networked personal computer (PC) or dedicated computer terminal near the telephone operator's desk can make this possible.

... or delegate scheduling duties UP

Spreading the scheduling duties out and delegating them downward to less-skilled staff works fine until a patient asks an unusual question or seems to have a more urgent medical need. When that happens, the patient gets transferred from the scheduling area to someone who has more medical training. Then, to make things more inconvenient and inefficient, the patient gets transferred back to the scheduler because the clinical person cannot, or is not allowed to, make an appointment for the patient.

Here's a way to reduce the handoffs and transfers and make the scheduling process runs smoother: delegate the scheduling responsibilities up, not just down and out.

Allow nurses and other clinically trained staff members to take over the scheduling process when patients ask complicated questions. Nurses and medical assistants with additional training can put their skills to work triaging patients, giving basic facts and judging the potential level of visit a patient may require. It will save the practice time and effort down the line to let these clinical staff members schedule appointments.

Doctor, may I schedule this patient?

One of the most inefficient scheduling practices routinely used by practices is to force schedulers to request permission to schedule appointments for certain diagnoses, certain specialists or for any urgent or same-day appointments.

This scheduling practice keeps an already distressed patient on hold while the scheduler tracks down a physician to review the case. When a physician demands that all new patients be pre-qualified before getting appointments, appointment schedulers must leave their workstations, wait for the physician to come out of an exam room, and ask for permission to schedule the new patient. While this is going on, the patient waits on hold. Telephone lines are tied up and other patients cannot schedule their appointments. It's a no-win situation.

Solution? Train scheduling staff to evaluate certain complaints or transfer all urgent/same-day appointment requests to a nurse who can triage and schedule appointments.

When physicians want to preapprove new patients, ask them to give schedulers some basic guidelines with prescribed questions and information, such as what insurance your practice accepts. Subspecialists worried about receiving referred patients with diagnoses they do not treat can create a preappointment screening process (see the Advanced Concept, "Preappointment Screening," at the end of this chapter).

Free your template hostages

When new physicians are hired by a practice, they often spend the first few days developing the ideal scheduling template. After years of dealing with whatever walked in the door of their residency program's clinic, new physicians feel refreshed by the notion that they can now see the patients they want to see. So these new physicians may spend hours setting up schedules that reflect their ideal number of consults, acute visits, new patients, and procedures.

Yet, after several months with their practice, it is common to find that the new physician's schedule is not very full. It may simply be because their practice is slow to mature. Or it could be a problem with the scheduling template. Physicians — particularly new ones who are not familiar with the patient population — tend to develop templates that meet *their* needs, but not those of their patients. Rigid scheduling templates can hold patients — and physician productivity — hostage.

Here's a good example of a template problem. A new (and not so busy) pediatrician received complaints from patients who said they had to wait for weeks to schedule well-child checks with her. What was happening was that when a parent asked for a well-child checkup, the scheduling staff dutifully looked for the next well-child checkup opening on the physician's template. Sometimes, parents had to wait many weeks, even though slots for acute or new patient visits remained open – and unused – during the current week. This new pediatrician had developed a template that was perfect for her but not her patients.

The scheduling template hostage crisis is often a problem for physicians who have recently joined a practice. Ask them to share scheduling preferences when they are recruited but don't let those preferences become barriers to productivity or patient access. Help newly recruited physicians build templates that reflect their needs as well as the needs and expectations of their new population of patients.

Empower schedulers to make decisions when a physician's supply of open appointments appears mismatched with patient demand. For example, let the scheduler set up a well-child visit in an acute-care slot if it appears that slot will go unfilled. When that happens, remind the physician to praise the scheduler's quick thinking instead of criticizing her for not following directions.

Meet with new physicians monthly. Ask them what's working and what's not with their schedule? Get another physician involved in these meetings to assure the new physician that his flexibility is critical to the practice's success.

Consider establishing the templates for all new physicians to your practice. Your practice knows best when it comes to the needs of your patients.

Remember, the ultimate goal of good scheduling is to see as many patients as possible, not to cling to a perfect-looking template that doesn't work.

Emergency calls

Suppose a 50-year-old patient calls your practice and asks for an appointment because she suddenly feels short of breath and has a sharp pain, first in her jaw and now in her upper back, but hasn't had any dental work recently and hasn't lifted anything heavy.

How would your scheduling staff respond? Would they take a message and tell the patient that the physician will call back? Or would they tell the patient to go to an emergency room because she is exhibiting signs of a heart attack?

It is critical to establish emergency protocols and to keep re-examining and updating them. Teach every member of your staff who answers telephones when to tell a patient to go directly to an emergency room or dial 911.

Creative ways to handle late arrivals

Patients who arrive late can frustrate well-honed scheduling protocols. One midwestern practice came up with a creative solution for late arrivals. Patients who arrived 15 (or more) minutes late for their appointment were given three options. They could either reschedule their appointment, wait to be worked in, or make an announcement to all of the patients in the waiting room that they were late and would be making all of the other patients (who had arrived on time) wait. In three years, no patient had chosen the last option.

Scheduling gaps should spur staff shifts

Gaps in schedules can cause problems, too. If there are fewer patients scheduled on Wednesday afternoons, the front office and nursing staff can use the time to return patients' telephone calls and catch up on the work left over from the previous week. That's a good breather, but it doesn't bring in any revenue to the practice.

Maybe there's a way to shift some of those staff members whose compensation and benefits are a big part of the practice's fixed costs to a busier part of the week to better assist patient flow and boost physician productivity.

How do you know which days are busier than others and, thus, need additional staffing to help solve patient flow problems? Staff may know intuitively which days are busier. Usually, Monday mornings are the busiest days. But you can do better than rely on intuition. Here's how.

Examine the weekly schedule for all of your physicians. Next, make a grid for an average week. Let's say your physicians have six hours set aside each day for direct patient contact – three hours in the morning and three hours in the afternoon. For example, 9:00 a.m. to Noon and 1:00 to 4:00 p.m.

 ...your practice has the "Monday mentality" syndrome when one of your staff tells an outsider:

"If you'd only been here on a Monday, you would have seen how hard we really work."

If the practice is open five days a week with morning and afternoon sessions each day, your chart will have five vertical columns with six boxes representing the hourly segments stacked under each column. Put a check mark into each box for each patient scheduled during that hour block. Then, add up all the check marks for each hour and for each morning and afternoon session. Next, calculate the average patient volume associated with each morning and afternoon session for each day. That is, the number of patients seen.

Now, look at the work schedules for all non-physicians on both the clinical and non-clinical sides of the practice. Apply those staffing ratios to each morning and afternoon session. If your practice is like most, the pattern you'll see emerge is that staffing numbers remain constant while the actual workload fluctuates from mornings to afternoons or from day to day.

Fluctuations in patient volume can be particularly profound in surgical practices where the outpatient practice is scheduled around operating room availability.

Let's look at an example (see following page):

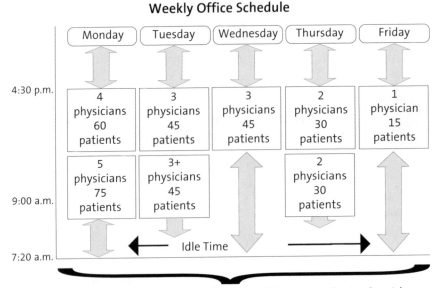

Weekly Office Schedule

75 full-time equivalent (FTE) staff Monday through Friday

The staffing/patient volume patterns shown are for a practice that quickly recognized that staffing (and the associated costs) remained constant while workloads varied considerably from session to session.

You can easily see a block of idle time from 7:30 to 8:30 a.m., as well as on Wednesday mornings. By making a few scheduling shifts, the result will be reduced idle time for employees, less frustration for the physician and shorter wait times for patients.

Don't assume your staff is idle during the blocks with lighter patient volume. They probably use that time to catch up on work caused by other inefficiencies in the practice, such as batching registration information, charge entry, telephone callbacks and so on. The lessons in this book can help you smooth out patient flow and keep your practice operating more efficiently.

Most specialties have seasonal fluctuations, and it's pretty easy to prepare for those. For example, most primary care practices know that flu season and school physicals bring increased volume to the practice during certain months. Specialists will notice other trends, too. That's why it can help to take last year's patient appointment data and plot it on out on a monthly basis.

For example:

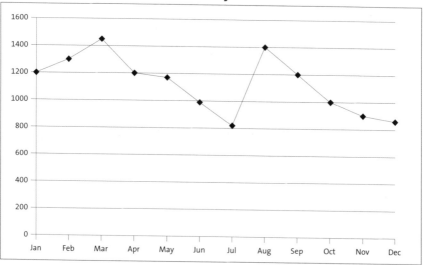

Encounters by Month

In order to make operations more efficient and smooth patient flow, this practice knows that it must increase its staffing levels in February, March and August by hiring part-time help. Ex-employees who are now stay-at-home parents, students who are interested in interning, and persons looking for per diem work are all options for part-timers. Part-timers are not only flexible – they're less expensive. Another way to smooth patient demand is to send notices about scheduling flu shots (fall/winter) and school physicals (summer) well in advance – or schedule special hours or days to take care of this extra demand.

Use better scheduling to contain facility cost

Removing scheduling gaps doesn't just reduce staffing costs; it also helps hold down facility and real estate expenses.

Practices often look for new space thinking that they have grown out of their existing space without really looking at the capacity. A simple exercise known as a capacity analysis might reveal that the problem is not square footage, it is inefficient scheduling. The clinical areas of a supposedly full facility are often in use less than 25 percent of the time.

Utilize the same analysis that you developed to evaluate staffing — but this time, you'll be looking at space. Take your patient encounters per hour, and divide them by the patient encounters that your facility can handle. So, if you have 6 exam rooms, see one patient every 60 minutes and have 5 patients between 10:00 and 11:00 a.m., your space utilization would be 83 percent during that hour.

Plot your space utilization by hour of the day in a chart to understand your daily capacity — and the opportunities to improve it.

Space Utilization by Hour of Day

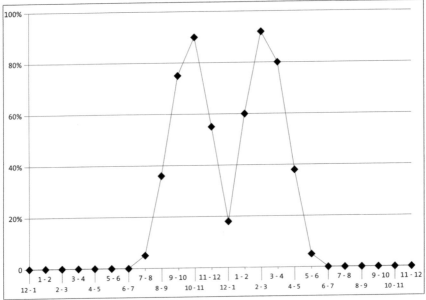

Your practice probably has more untapped capacity than you realize. Maybe better scheduling can allow you to put off an expensive facility expansion or a move to a larger office.

Most physicians spend between 5 percent and 10 percent of their revenue stream on real estate. That's four to five times what they spend on information technology and telecommunications. But what most practices forget is that their building investment offers capacity 24 hours a day, seven days a week. Of course, you won't get many patients to schedule their appointments at 2:00 a.m., but here are some ways to get more out of your facility:

Adjust schedules for seasonal variations. School physicals make August a busy month for family medicine and pediatric practices. Many allergists' offices seem deserted in July. Surgical practices can expect fewer patients around holidays. Look at the number of office visits your practice received each for that past year. Are there seasonal variations in your practice? Maybe you can balance the use of your facility by opening the doors on Saturdays during busy months, or by going to schools and worksites to conduct physicals instead of using office space.

Examine a typical week to find the busy days. Maybe you're stuck with too much facility downtime on certain days. Mondays are booked solid but your practice, like many, has a light schedule on Friday afternoons. You like to wind down before the weekend but does that also mean that some patients have to wait longer to see their doctor or wait until Monday to get a prescription filled?

Review surgery schedules. Keeping your facility at optimal capacity may also be a function of scheduling the physician's time at the hospital or surgery center. If office hours become secondary to operating room time, then physicians are left holding the bag for expensive office space that isn't being used.

Analyze how your office is really used. Yes, you have office hours posted, but is your facility really in full use during those hours? Most practices don't start seeing patients until 20 to 30 minutes after the office doors open. Often, just one or two patients are seen during the last quarter hour of the day. Your practice might be jammed from 9:00 to 11:00 a.m., slow during midday, and hopping again from 1:30 to 3:30 p.m. Are you really out of space when most of your exam rooms sit empty for two or more hours during your posted hours?

Use your capacity analysis to make a difference. For example, alternate lunch schedules among physicians so that exam rooms always remain full. Schedule the day's first appointments to start 15 to 30 minutes before the physician's posted hours. A medical assistant can greet and process the day's first patients so that they are waiting in the exam room when the physician walks in to the office. Consider extending hours. A growing trend is for medical practices to stay open from 7:00 a.m. to 7:00 p.m. two to four days a week. An extended schedule can transform six to eight hours of a day's worth of capacity into 10 to 12 hours – and it doesn't cost you any more rent.

Before you consider any facility expansions or relocate to gain more clinical space, make sure you're getting full use out of your current facility.

Give the patient a heads up

Do your patients and your practice a big favor by training schedulers to let patients know exactly what they should bring to their appointment (e.g., copayment, radiology films, forms, etc.).

The scheduler also should give patients a best estimate of how long to expect their appointment to take on average. That is, "Periodic physicals for your age group take 30 minutes on average in our practice." Repeat this information during the appointment reminder call, if one is made, but make sure it's the same information. Many automated reminder systems can be customized. Reducing the surprise factor will create a more informed patient.

Smoother communication smoothes schedule delays

Take a lesson from the airlines: keeping customers in the dark when there are delays just makes them madder.

Medical emergencies can cause a physician's scheduled patients to wait longer. But there are good and bad ways to deliver this news. When an emergency arises and a physician can't see scheduled patients on time, take these steps:

Ask physicians to notify the office immediately. Make sure the news gets passed on. The clinical support staff often hear about a physician's delay but forget – or not think – to let the front office know. The front office bears the brunt of patients' frustrations, so keep them in the loop.

Require that a member of the clinical support team, whenever possible, deliver the news to waiting patients. Patients may perceive the nurse as the physician's spokesperson, but see the receptionist as only a gatekeeper.

Immediately give delayed patients the choice to reschedule or wait. People tend to feel less put-upon when they have a choice. If necessary, bring extra staff to the front office to help with rescheduling.

Ask the receptionist to telephone scheduled patients that may be affected by the delay. Give patients who have not yet arrived the opportunity to reschedule if it appears that the delay may be lengthy.

Delayed physicians should deliver the news, too. Ask delayed physicians to step into the reception area when they arrive to apologize for the delay, thank the patients for waiting and indicate that they will be with them as soon as possible.

You can never tell when a medical emergency will happen, but you can try to alleviate patients' frustrations over these inevitable delays.

Things to consider about handling delays

I once observed a physician handle an emergency-related delay with great skill. He went into the waiting room to apologize and explain to patients that a medical emergency had caused the delay. His staff had made the announcement earlier, but the two minutes it took for the physician to tell his patients personally had a great calming effect on the entire reception area — even for other physician's patients. Handled differently, the same situation could have created an uproar, rather than roomful of loyal patients.

No-shows happen for a reason

No-shows are the bane of smooth scheduling. But there will always be no-shows. The questions are: how many can you expect, how can you prevent them from disrupting your day and how can you reduce their frequency?

What is the average no-show rate for medical practices? It can range from as low as 5 percent to as high as 60 percent of all appointments. What makes the difference in handling no-shows is how your practice deals with them.

Here are some things that may cause your no-show rates to be higher than expected:

The patient-physician relationship. Practices in which physicians routinely rotate, including residency clinics and locum tenens, tend to have higher no-show rates. So do clinics in which physicians rotate through different practice sites throughout the week and ask patients to follow them to different sites. Patients may get confused about which site to visit or find one practice site much less convenient. The less loyalty patients have to the practice, the more likely they will be no-shows.

Payer mix and your hours. Some patients may not have reliable transportation, dependable childcare or enough flexibility at their workplace to schedule appointments during your practice's regular hours.

The amount of time to next appointment. Practices that schedule appointments 60 days out or more will find that patients are more likely to make alternate plans. They also may find other physicians who can get them in sooner, they get better in the meantime or they just forget.

Specialty of physician. Psychiatry and certain other specialties may experience higher no-show rates. Some patients may perceive that there is a stigma in having to seek help from certain types of specialists. On the opposite extreme, specialties such as pediatric neurosurgery will not likely find no-shows to be a problem.

Managing no-shows

Good data can help a practice manage its no-shows instead of letting them do the managing.

If you figure that your practice's no-show rate is 10 percent and your physician has slots to see, say, 20 patients per day, then expand your scheduling template to 22 slots. If your data are reliable, you can expect that, on the average day, two patients won't show up. Commonly known as overbooking, this practice is widespread but don't let it prevent you from trying to become more efficient. That is, don't rely on overbooking as the only way to increase the practice's productivity.

Instead, consider these 10 strategies to reduce your no-shows altogether:

Improve your relationship with patients. A strong relationship with patients strengthens the commitment they feel toward your practice. One way to build this bond is to send birthday cards to patients (use the date of birth from your registration database) or greeting cards at the holidays.

Create stronger nurse-patient relationships. Assign nurses to patients, especially those who have chronic conditions and who make many return visits to the practice. It may also help increase patient compliance. Print business cards for nurses to distribute to patients.

Provide timely access. Evaluate your time to the next available appointment. The average number of days patients must wait for an appointment with a physician, according to the American Medical Association, is 9.5 days.

Knowing the access time for your own specialty and your own market is more critical than knowing the national average, especially if your practice has competitors. To find out what's happening with wait times in your area, monitor your competition by contacting them to see when their next available appointment is for a new patient. Don't actually schedule an appointment; just call the competing practice(s) as a "new patient" to ask about appointment availability.

Consider using advanced access scheduling. Track walk-in and same-day appointment requests so you can balance these requests with anticipated no-shows. Adjust hours of operation, if possible, to include more early morning, noon hour, late afternoon and weekend appointment hours.

Do internal monitoring. Track your no-show statistics by physician, insurance company, day of week, month and by practice site to determine if overbooking is really necessary — and when. Consider the effect of your practice location on the no-show rate — does one office site have more no-shows than another? Keeping tabs on no shows — particularly those that are due to patient access problems — also helps your practice know when to recruit new physicians.

Establish a policy for repeat no-shows. Either decline to schedule patients who have missed several appointments (i.e., treat them as walk-ins instead) or discharge them from your practice.

Remind patients. Make appointment reminder calls 48 hours before the visit. Reminding patients of appointments plays a key role in reducing no-shows. Consider buying a telephony product that can automatically make reminder calls; many new systems can read your schedule (if it's automated) and may be programmed with one of your staff member's voices.

If telephone calls or sending postcard reminders don't work, try collecting pager and cell phone numbers so you can contact your more "wired" patients. E-mail can be used, but only with the written permission of the patient, particularly if the e-mail account resides at the patient's workplace. HIPAA rules do not forbid e-mail reminders, but they do require you to take reasonable measures to protect patient confidentiality. Think twice before sending bulk e-mails. And remember, employers have a right to look at their employee's e-mails so don't let your e-mail reminder efforts compromise a patient's wishes to keep to medical information confidential from his employer. (See Chapter 3, "Telephones," for more information.)

Call back to confirm. Ask new patients or those getting procedures to call you back to confirm that they received your appointment reminder and are planning to keep the appointment. The reminder notice – recording or postcard – warns the patient that the appointment will be rescheduled and the time slot given to someone else unless they call back by a certain time. If they don't call to confirm, pull from a waiting list of patients who want to get in sooner and slot them in.

Most practices only require callbacks from new patients, for certain procedures or other expensive visits. As with no-show charges and other policies, give patients advance warning of this requirement in writing and verbally when they schedule their appointments. Make sure you have enough staff and telephone capacity to handle the extra incoming telephone calls this policy may generate. Although I discuss ways to reduce the costs of incoming telephone calls in Chapter 3, "Telephones," the call that helps produce a paying patient is always worth taking.

Reminders

THINGS TO CONSIDER

✓ Keep the appointment fresh – don't make calls more than 72 hours in advance of the appointment.

✓ Keep communications confidential – send letters in a sealed envelope. Don't put the name of your specialty on the envelope – just the last name of your physician(s).

✓ Do not leave a voice mail or answering machine message that mentions the nature of the patient's visit.

✓ Ask new patients if you can leave future appointment reminders on their answering machines, voice mail or with others who might answer the telephone for them. Make sure their consent is in writing and included with appropriate Health Insurance Portability and Accountability (HIPAA) documentation.

✓ Use the 15-minute rule when you can't confirm every appointment. Identify which patients may need longer (than 15 minutes) or more complicated visits; make sure to send them reminders and seek confirmations.

✓ Consider gathering cell phone numbers and/or pagers during patient registration to reach patients regarding their reminders.

✓ Automate the appointment reminder process to ensure that all patients are reminded – and to redirect your staff effort to greeting, answering telephones, and other important front desk functions.

Ask patients to confirm appointments

Faced with a 50% no-show rate, Midtown Specialty Practice uses this script:

"Our new policy on appointments requires you to confirm your appointment at least 48-hours in advance so please call us at 123-4567 to secure your appointment time."

The practice gives patients at least a day to retrieve and respond to the message. Their no-show rate has dropped to less than 5 percent.

Don't schedule too far in advance. A scheduling template that extends many months into the future can increase no-show rates because patients will likely forget about a routine follow-up appointment that is scheduled 12 months in advance. The patient may have made other plans by the time she receives your appointment reminder call or postcard.

To reduce no-shows and cancellations when visits must be scheduled several months out, put those appointments into a manual or automatic queue. The queue can trigger a printed or telephonic reminder notice to the patient six to eight weeks before the scheduled appointment. Require the patient to confirm the appointment.

Charge patients. Charge a nominal no-show fee (unless insurance companies forbid it in their contracts with you) to patients who do not show up for appointments and fail to cancel.

Inevitably, even the practice with the most compliant patients will have a no-show. People are forgetful. No matter how well you manage no-shows, it's still important to have a mechanism in place to track them. Tracking no-shows is important from two perspectives: patient compliance (so you can follow up with the patient) and billing and collections (so you match your charges to the services provided).

From a compliance perspective, you want to follow up with a patient who visited your practice to receive news of a malignant tumor or some other important medical information. Remember, it's your responsibility to care for your patients even if they sometimes miss an appointment. Work with your malpractice carrier to determine the best possible route to follow up with patients if this is a problem for your practice.

No-shows have an impact on billing and collections because you must be sure to bill all of the patients who present at the practice. Without knowing who did not show up for their appointments, you cannot track the patients who did indeed come.

More on charging for no-shows

No-shows cost your practice money through lost opportunity. For years, practice management experts have debated whether it was worth it to charge patients who missed scheduled appointments. With practice overhead costs rising every year, your practice may soon join the growing number of practices that do charge for no-shows.

Typical no-show charges range from $15 to $25. You may end up waiving many of these charges – patients may have legitimate transportation or childcare problems that occur at the last minute. Counsel them on what to do the next time it happens. Billing patients for not showing up for appointments does get their attention but capturing these nominal charges is not the primary goal; it's reducing the rate of no-shows.

If you do decide to charge for no-shows, be sure to communicate the new policy in advance to all patients. Send them a letter, post signs in the office and ask schedulers to remind patients of the policy when they make appointments.

Most insurance companies, including Medicare, will not pay for no-show charges, although some insurance companies may allow your practice to charge the patients (their beneficiaries) directly. Check with the insurance companies to ensure that your no-show strategy is in compliance with their rules.

You can't bill them if you can't find them

Don't even try to charge for no-shows if your practice serves an indigent population or other hard-to-reach populations. You'll spend more on mailing bills for the $15 no-show charge to wrong addresses than you could possibly hope to collect. Also stop billing patients for not showing up if the cost of doing so draws precious human or financial resources away from your billing office's more important and lucrative task of following up on insurance claims that are pending or have been denied.

Physicians can be no-shows, too

Patients aren't the only no shows who disrupt the practice's business. Sometimes, physicians cancel appointments because they want leisure time or want to attend other functions at the last minute. We tend to use code words like "bumping" the appointments, but whatever term you choose to use, this behavior is hazardous to practice productivity and customer service.

Try this five-step exercise to head off physician bumps:

Step One: Track "bumped" appointments separately from patient no-shows.

Step Two: Include "bumped" appointments in the regular monthly performance reports you prepare for the group's physician owners.

Step Three: Use actual not scheduled patient visits to compute physician productivity. Using scheduled visits allows the physicians who habitually cancel appointments to receive just as much productivity credit as colleagues who don't routinely "bump" their patients.

Step Four: Track the administrative burden that having to cancel and reschedule appointments places on employees. Figure out how long it takes to schedule and reschedule the typical appointment;

multiply by the number of physician-canceled appointments in the previous month; and multiply by the hourly wage plus benefits of the staffer who schedules appointments. Let's look at an example:

Average time to schedule an appointment: 10 minutes

Average time to reschedule an appointment: 15 minutes

Average number of physician-cancelled appointments during past month: 43

Average hourly wage (including benefits) for schedulers: $12

Average cost of rescheduling each appointment: $3 ($12/15 minutes or 0.25 hours)

Cost of rescheduling 43 appointments past month: $129

If the practice annualized its data to include one year, the cost would be $1,548.

But, wait a minute. Does the cost of the medical assistant for that afternoon's bumped schedule disappear? Of course not. Since most of the practice's costs are fixed (see Chapter 10, "Fundamental Financials"), the canceled clinics result in a loss of revenue (opportunity cost) for the afternoon's lost appointments.

Let's look at the opportunity cost for cancelled appointments:

Average contribution per patient: $45

Cost of losing the 43 patient visits last month: $1,935

If the practice annualized its data to include one year, the cost would be $23,220.

Nearly $25,000 lost on canceled clinics in one year! Moreover, this does not take into account the fact that having their appointments canceled and rescheduled is one of the fastest ways to make patients unhappy. Yet, it is a factor that is almost entirely under the practice's control.

Step Five: Establish a "bumped" appointment policy. Present your lost opportunity computations for bumped appointments to the practice's physician owners. They may wish to allow physicians to only "bump" patients six weeks or more in advance. Once the appointment is less than six weeks away, the policy would allow changes only for emergencies. If your practice continues to experience a problem with bumped appointments, ask the practice's board of directors to require physicians who cancel appointments for personal reasons to personally call every affected patient to apologize and to reschedule.

CASE STUDIES

Southeast Surgical Partners cuts "bumps"

There were so many canceled clinics at Southeast Surgical Partners that it took almost 40 hours a week in combined staff time just to manage all the tasks involved in contacting patients to reschedule clinics that physicians had canceled. The administrator calculated that the cost of physicians canceling appointments for non-emergency reasons was almost $30,000 a year. Once alerted to how much Southeast Surgical Partners was spending to reschedule clinics, the physician leaders introduced administrative policies similar to those described in the "Physicians can be no-shows, too" section. Since then, the "bump" rate at Southeast Surgical Partners has been cut by 80 percent. The reduction in staff time dedicated to this rescheduling function was worth $24,000.

Surgery scheduling

For surgical practices, the scheduling of surgeries is a critical component of practice operations. All of the scheduling techniques described thus far have related to office appointments; I'll now spend some time on surgery scheduling.

Surgery scheduling is an essential process that must be conducted in a timely manner to ensure that both the patient's and the surgeon's time are respected. It is important for the individual scheduling the appointment to know the physician's individual scheduling preferences (based on the duration of the surgery).

The pre-authorization or pre-certification process is typically coordinated with the scheduling of a surgery. Although the specifics of the process depend on the medical specialty and the insurance companies involved, some processes are standard. They include:

Consent to treat: The patient must consent in writing to have the surgery performed. Typically, the physician presents the consent form for signature in the exam room. However, the surgery scheduler must always check that this important form has been completed and is attached to the patient's file. Consent forms are regulated by each state, so be sure to check with your state medical society to make sure that you're using the right one.

Schedule: The time and date of the surgery are determined based on the surgeon's calendar. Then the hospital or outpatient surgery facility is contacted to put the patient on the operating room schedule. Any required pre- or post-op arrangements should be made at this time.

Pre-admission: The scheduler must ensure that the hospital or outpatient surgery has all of the appropriate diagnostic test results, a clearance physical and/or any other clinical and administrative requirements required by the facility.

Pre-authorization/certification: The insurance company must be contacted on the telephone or online to request authorization to perform the surgery. The scheduler usually makes this contact, although sometimes a nurse or the billing office may be responsible for this component. Typically, the insurance company will request some background information about the diagnosis and treatment, so the staff member handling the details of this step should have clinical training or a solid clinical knowledge base.

Financial responsibility: Practices attuned to patient collections take the opportunity to introduce the patient to his financial responsibility during the scheduling process. During the contact with the insurance company about the pre-authorization, the scheduler asks for details of the patient's financial responsibility to include the deductible (what, if any, is remaining), coinsurance and any other responsibility. A worksheet is developed for the patient that outlines his responsibility. Many practices also ask for some – if not all – of the patient's portion of the payment before the surgery.

At all stages in communicating with others (primary care physician, hospital and insurance company), it is important for the surgeon's staff to record the date, time and the person(s) with whom they speak. If problems arise, this information can be invaluable in determining who said what, when and to whom.

Keep track of surgery scheduling

Develop a single form to track all information involved in scheduling surgery. If one person is assigned to conduct the process for the practice and has a particular method, it is essential that someone else be cross-trained in how to schedule surgery. You don't want the process to be put on hold or fall apart if the individual who normally handles the task goes on vacation, takes sick leave or resigns. Problems that occur at this stage, such as a missing authorization or consent form, can come back to haunt the practice.

Having a single form (see example) in which all of the required information and communication regarding the surgery is placed can help this function move smoothly, efficiently and accurately.

Surgery Scheduling Template

Date:	Initials:
Patient's Name:	DOB
SS#	Phone (h) (w)
Address:	
City/State/Zip code:	
Referring MD:	Phone: Notified? / /
Will they do H&P? Y / N	Will they schedule H&P? Y / N
PCP:	Phone:
Diagnosis?	
Procedure(s)?	
Scheduled for: Date: / /	Time: Hospital:
Scheduled by:	(hospital) (office)
Anesthesia:	
Pre-Op:	
Patient Instructions:	
Patient Notified? Y / N / / (date)	
Insurance:	
Policy No.	Group No.
Patient Financial Responsibility:	
Deductible met? Y / N	If not, what amount remains?
Coinsurance? Y / N	
Total balance:	
Amount collected from patient?	Amount on payment plan?
Precertification Needed? Y / N	
Obtained by: (office)	(insurance co.) / / (date)
PRE-CERT NO:	
Notes:	

Things to Consider about OR Scheduling

For surgical practices that can never seem to get enough operating room (OR) time, ask your hospital(s) if they offer "block scheduling" in the OR. In this arrangement, the hospital provides a guarantee for your surgeons to have full use of its OR for a specific block of time (for example, 7:00 a.m. to 5:00 p.m. every Tuesday). The advantage is that instead of managing your OR day around the hospital's schedule, your physicians get full use of a dedicated time block. This allows your practice to manage its time better and create a schedule that maximizes the surgeon's time.

Appointment recalls

Appointment recall systems prove valuable in assuring timely and appropriate care management. Appointment recalls are the practice's method of tracking the next visit(s) that the physician has recommended. For example, if a patient receives a well-woman checkup in November and a follow-up visit for a small mole is recommended in March, the practice should record, track and communicate with the patient in February to remind her of the follow-up appointment needed in March.

Although manual recall logs, which record all appointments or other reminders in date order, are the traditional method, automating the recall system is a timesaving measure. Many practice management systems and electronic medical records can conduct the recall process by automatically sending appointment notices telephonically or in writing to patients. Alternatively, a recall list can be generated to prompt a physician to review a patient's medical records to decide if a recall is appropriate.

Scheduling is the key to managing patient flow. Combining the physician's work style with creative processes will leave your practice – and your patients – satisfied.

Preappointment screening

Does your subspecialty practice focus on a narrow field of clinical care? Do your specialists receive too many referrals for patients whose diagnoses lie outside their area of expertise? Maybe preappointment screening is for you.

Preappointment screening is the process of screening calls for appointments prior to scheduling them to determine whether they are appropriate for your practice. For example, if you are an otolaryngology practice that focuses only on sinus surgery, then a patient calling about a hearing problem would not be given an appointment. Instead, he would be referred to another otolaryngologist or sent back to the referring physician for her advice.

Subspecialists who wish to screen patient appointments should include education for referring physicians and patients self-referring or seeking a second opinion. Annoying or confusing the referring physician or the patient is the major risk of preappointment screening.

For referring physicians, talk to your primary referral sources. Tell them what your group of subspecialists handles best, what they can't or don't want to handle, what kind of access to expect for referred patients and where to refer patients who don't fit your practice's areas of expertise. Describe your physicians' areas of expertise on written materials and on your Web site.

For patients who are self-referring or wishing a second opinion, outline concrete instructions about what information to submit and to whom. Be clear about what tests, notes, physical characteristics, and so forth you need to make a decision.

The entire appointment process – information gathering, review and the setting or denying of the appointment – should be handled in a short, defined period of time. Empower one or two individuals to make those decisions. Don't route patients or referring physicians through an extensive and frustrating web of gatekeepers and processes. Give a scheduling flow chart or algorithm to the staff member who is responsible for screening appointments.

If you are a group, it's important to note that sub-specializing may create a problem. If your practice gets so specialized that it will not handle any of your specialty area's general issues, this creates an opportunity for someone to capture market share. If your practice starts to appear too exclusive, a competing group of specialists may develop a relationship with your referring physicians. It is becoming more common to see generalist groups seize the opportunity – and your referral stream – by adding subspecialty expertise to their group practice.

Preappointment screening can backfire if your process of information gathering, clinical review and communication about the appointment itself is too cumbersome and time-consuming. That's why you must monitor this process carefully.

If managed effectively, preappointment screening can be very useful to subspecialists who do not wish to handle all of the general issues that their specialty's name implies – and it can mean getting the right care to the patient more efficiently.

Physician supply and patient demand

How do you determine when is the right time to recruit another physician? Measuring supply and demand can give you a quick – and accurate – answer. Determining when patient demand exceeds your supply of physicians is a complex concept, but one that is essential to managing your operations. In essence, it's the question that you should ask when you notice signs that your practice isn't keeping up with patient demand, such as a steadily increasing time to next available appointment. Before you jump into the recruiting process – or ever worse, sit back and do nothing, a simple access and productivity analysis can make a difficult determination fairly easy.

Create a chart to measure access and productivity. Make the x-axis the number of days to your next available new patient appointment, and the y-axis relative value units (RVUs) per half-day clinic. Obtain national benchmarks for these data points for your specialty.

Plot the data for each physician in your practice, as well as the national benchmarks. A sample chart is presented for a urology practice with four physicians.

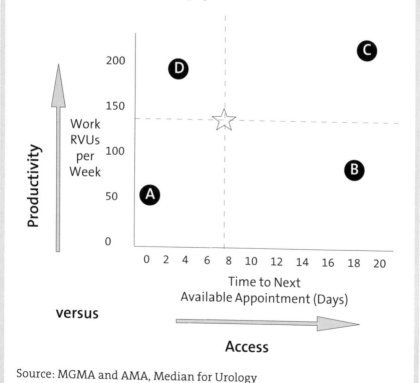

Source: MGMA and AMA, Median for Urology

The results are simple, but telling:

If most of your physicians are in the upper left quadrant (like Physician D), you have good access and good productivity.

If some of your physicians are in the lower right quadrant (like Physician B), you have poor access and poor productivity. This is a problem, but not one that recruiting another physician can help with. Instead, find ways to make those particular physicians more efficient. Maybe they need more staff, smoother work habits or a little motivation. If they are near retirement, displaying this data may be the impetus to exit.

If there is a physician in the lower left quadrant (like Physician A), you had better hope that it's a new physician. Good access and poor productivity are characteristics of a practice that has yet to mature. If the physician has been in practice for many years, it's time to find out why he or she is unproductive and not in demand. You may have a real problem on your hands that recruiting won't help at all.

If most are in the upper right quadrant (like Physician C), you need to recruit – soon. Your physicians are highly productive but patients have to wait to get in to see them. Since you've maximized productivity, access will continue to be a problem. If you don't get another physician or midlevel provider in soon, a backlog – and all of the inefficiencies that stem from it – will develop soon.

Measuring physician supply and patient demand on this productivity/access grid is an easy way to get the answer to the very complex question of if and when to recruit another physician.

Group visits

Group visits can boost collections and patient satisfaction. During group visits, physicians can see 6 to 12 patients at once. Instead of a traditional 10- to 20-minute encounter with one patient (four hours to see 12 patients), a physician can see 12 patients in just 60 to 90 minutes.

Group visits work well for certain types of patients who need certain services. But look around. There may be many of these patients in your practice. In a group visit for diabetic patients, the physician can explain the condition to 10 patients at once – instead of 10 different times during the week. This leaves more time for patients to discuss more individualized issues during one-on-one visits with their physician.

Since group visits can include midlevel providers, such as dieticians, patients get more education from different experts. Many patients find group visits supportive because they are with others who have similar complaints or conditions. Sometimes, the supportive environment allows physicians to address sensitive concerns that a patient might feel too embarrassed to bring up during a one-on-one visit.

Rightly so, group visits may raise concerns about patient privacy, as well they should. Since patients may ask questions or provide comments in a group — and other patients will hear about their medical condition — make sure that your practice has a confidentiality waiver agreement in place.

Words of wisdom about confidentiality in group visits

Patients have expectations of privacy and confidentiality when they visit your practice, regardless of whether it's for a group visit or a one-on-one visit with their physician. Even though you ask group-visit patients to sign confidentiality waivers, advise them that your practice respects patient privacy and they should, too. Tell group-visit patients that they are not expected to share with the group any share personal information that they would want only their doctor — and no one else — to know.

Tell group-visit patients that anything they learn about individual group members should not leave the room. And remind patients that respect for the privacy and opinions of others is what makes the group visit work. Finally, and most importantly, never force a patient to have a group visit in lieu of a one-on-one visit. Offer it as an option, and let the patient make the choice.

Types of group visits

- **Drop-in medical group appointments (DIGMAs).** Invite patients to "drop-in" for an office visit at a specific time. The only criteria for participation is to be on the physician's panel. In this approach, a physician and another nonphysician health professional lead the visit. Since the group meets at the same time and day each week, patients may drop in when they choose. However, ask patients to register in advance so that their charts are pulled before they arrive. This type of visit works well for patients who have chronic diseases and have a lot of information and support needs.

- **Educational sessions.** An OB/GYN practice might provide or host a childbirth class. An infectious disease practice might provide or host an educational session for international travelers. These courses generally are scheduled in advance and often led by nurses.

- **Cooperative health care clinics (CHCCs).** Scheduled visits that include an educational component but which are focused on helping patients meet certain criteria, such as boosting dietary compliance for diabetics. Developed by John Scott, MD, for his geriatric patients, this model has expanded to include other patients with chronic diseases (e.g., congestive heart failure) or other shared situations (e.g., pediatric well-child visits). CHCCs often involve a multidisciplinary team but are led by a physician.

Group visits are easy to schedule. Here's how: Choose diabetes, arthritis or another common condition shared by many of your practice's patients. Or select a type of mandatory checkup such as nine-month well-child visits. Ask up to 15 patients if they'd like to have their next visit in a group setting. Explain the concept to them face-to-face, in a brief phone call or write a statement detailing the benefits of a group visit. Emphasize that their privacy is protected and how they can benefit from interacting with other patients and, if applicable, the other clinicians who will assist.

The group visit should be offered as an option or an enhancement to one-on-one care. Ask interested patients to sign a statement describing the visit's protocols and return the form to you to indicate they will attend the session. From your pool of 15 patients, expect that 10 to 12 will show up.

Register the patients prior to the visit, and pull their charts ahead of time. During the session, ask two medical assistants to record each patient's vitals and chief complaints privately in nearby exam rooms, just as they would during a regular patient visit.

Next, gather the patients in a conference to hear the physician present a five- to 10-minute presentation on relevant medical issues. Then, medical assistants escort the patients to exam rooms one-by-one for their physical exam by the physician.

While patients wait their turn to see the physician, they can ask questions of an educator – your dietician, for example – or talk to other patients who have similar problems. A medical assistant can take blood or complete other orders during this time, too.

After completing the physicals or exams, the physician returns to the group to answer patients' general questions and wraps up the session.

At the time of publication of this book, there are no CPT codes for group visits. However, the CPT Advisory Committee is taking this new means of delivering services under advisement. In the meantime, some practices are billing evaluation and management (E&M) codes for patients attending the group visit. If you're billing an E&M code, make sure that all of the requirements for the code are met and documented, and check with your insurance companies to make sure they accept that a group setting meets the requirements of an E&M encounter.

Group visits are a "win-win" for your practice and your patients. It doesn't hurt to try them – it only takes a little time and effort for your practice to test the concept.

Group Visits

- ❑ What will the criteria be for the group?
- ❑ When will the group be held?
- ❑ How will we inform our patients?
- ❑ How will we make the appointments?
- ❑ Where will we hold the group visit?
- ❑ Do we need adjoining exam rooms?
- ❑ Who will "host" the visit?
- ❑ When and how will we pull the patients' charts?
- ❑ How and when will we register the patients?
- ❑ How will we document the visit?
- ❑ How will we bill for the visit?

ADVANCED CONCEPT

Express clinics

Some years ago, many practices decided that extending office hours in the evening would be a great idea for their working patients. Evening hours are great for patients, but many practices have trouble convincing employees and physicians to staff evening clinics. Many practices must pay premium wages or overtime to maintain their evening hours. With more physicians who want to be home by 5:30 p.m. to see their child's baseball game or fix dinner for the family, some practices have discontinued evening hours.

Is there an alternative to serve patients who must be at work from 9:00 a.m. to 5:00 p.m.? Express clinics in the morning are filling that need.

In particular, pediatric practices have embraced the concept by offering early morning clinic hours for sick child visits with no appointments needed.

The clinics are popular. Parents get fast help for their sick child and still get to work on time. Since parents know that their child will be seen early in the morning, physicians get fewer non-emergency calls in the middle of the night. The practice increases revenue because physicians usually cannot bill insurance for giving advice over the phone, no matter how late at night it is. With express clinics, the patients are seen face-to-face. In addition to being a billable event, patient care is improved with actual physical contact with the patient.

Express clinics aren't just for pediatric practices; they can work for many other specialties. For example, internal medicine practices can open early to serve patients suffering sudden colds, flu symptoms or rashes. Allergy practices can designate special hours for patients who need regular maintenance shots.

To run a successful express clinic, you must carefully match your practice's physician supply with your patient demand – a difficult task. Above all, you must remain flexible.

Here's how to do a rough estimate of your patient population's demand for an express clinic, the number of staff you'll need and the hours the clinic should remain open to achieve its full potential.

- For a month, evaluate the calls your physicians on call receive at night. How many calls come from patients (or their caregivers) whose acute problems were not emergencies? How many calls were about concerns that could have been treated several hours later (e.g., a 2:00 a.m. call treated in the office at 7:00 a.m.)?

- Review your nurse call logs to determine the average number of patients who call in afternoons or evenings to make appointments for an acute visit the following morning. These patients may also want to go to your express clinics, thus opening up more acute slots during the middle of the day. If you want your practice to grow, you could also consider opening new patient appointment slots to replace these during the day.

- Use the call analyses to estimate the number of visits you would receive if you opened an express clinic. For example, if you receive 15 calls a night about non-emergent issues, and 10 of them were concerns that would have normally been addressed in the office had the patient called during the day, then anticipate 8 to 10 express clinic appointments. Add to this number an estimate of the patients who call in the afternoon asking for an acute visit the following morning. If you think that they'd prefer a 7:00 a.m. slot versus a 9:00 a.m. slot, then they're candidates for your express clinic.

- Multiply your practice's average revenue per encounter by your volume estimate. The result is the express clinic's estimated daily revenue. To get your average revenue per encounter, take your collections from the year prior and divide this number by your encounters for that year. It will likely be in the range of $50 to $200 per encounter.

- Use the volume estimates to determine the hours and staff for your express clinic. If you estimate that only two patients will show up, start the express clinic 30 minutes before existing office hours, and have the medical assistant and receptionist come 30 minutes earlier than regular office hours. If you think that 10 patients will take advantage of your express clinic, you may need more staff and physicians. Replicate your staffing from the "regular" day, but don't overstaff the express clinic. Try using staggered staff and physician schedules so you can operate the express clinic with little to no additional overhead.

- Re-evaluate after a few weeks. If demand is higher than you estimated, then consider expanding hours or increasing the number of physicians. Try creating express clinics for subsets of your patients. For example, an OB/GYN practice might control demand by opening an express clinic for prenatal patients. Or, if there not enough patients with acute needs to fill the appointment slots, consider opening the clinic up to other types of appointments, such as physicals, consultations or new patients. Before you change the model, however, note that the express clinic will be slow at first as your patients learn about this new option.

No matter how carefully you analyze appointment demand, expect that there will be days when an unexpected flood of patients shows up – or no one at all.

Flexibility is the key to your express clinic's success. Your physicians may object at first but remind them that they are doing the same work – but for free – in the middle of the night while on call.

The best part of an express clinic is that you can try it once, and return to your normal hours if it doesn't work.

Chapter 5

REGISTRATION

Key Chapter Lessons

> Recognize the tools to create an effective workstation at registration

> Understand the value of registration in the billing process

> Learn five ways to pre-register your patients

> Examine the process of insurance verification

> Learn the key components of site registration for new and established patients

> Familiarize yourself with check-in requirements

> Evaluate and find alternatives for the sign-in list

> Develop a system to communicate the patient's arrival to the clinical team

> Evaluate your check-in process

Advanced Concepts

> Exam Room Registration

Registration checklist

- ❏ Is the receptionist prepared for patients to check-in?

- ❏ Are patients greeted by name at the time of arrival?

- ❏ Do patients feel recognized and their presence welcomed? Or does the staff make patients feel like they are an interruption or annoyance?

- ❏ Are patients greeted with enthusiasm, respect and concern? Or is it likely that patients are made to feel "like a number" or "like a diagnosis"?

- ❏ Is the receptionist on a telephone headset in addition to handling reception duties?

- ❏ How are you ensuring the collection of accurate information?

- ❏ Would your reception area pass a critical review? Is it clean, neat and quiet?

- ❏ Are reading materials in the reception area current and appropriate?

- ❏ Are patients regularly seen within 20 minutes of their appointment time and presentation?

- ❏ Are patients likely to agree that their privacy and confidentiality were protected?

- ❏ Does the person escorting patients walk with the patients in order to accompany them to the exam room or does that person call out patients' names from the doorway?

- ❏ Are patients asked to provide information that they have already provided to someone else in your practice?

- ❏ Are delays communicated to patients promptly and effectively?

© 2003 Larch/Woodcock/Walker. Used with permission.

"The patient has arrived! Now what?"

Having scheduled a patient and reminded him when to come and what to bring, your next contact with the patient is at check-in. As with telephones and scheduling, this function offers many opportunities to make your practice more efficient.

Check-in should be quick, efficient and relatively painless for both the patient and the practice. Attention to detail at this early point in the patient flow process will save your staff and physicians considerable work down the line. Attention to courtesy will keep "patients patient" if physicians are running late. Most importantly, courtesy will keep patients willing to come back to your practice instead of another one.

This chapter will examine ways to streamline the functions within the check-in process, including pre-registration, registration and sign in.

Don't make registration a source of pain

Does your receptionist greet patients by avoiding eye contact, pointing to a clipboard and mumbling, "sign in"? If so, your practice is saying, in effect, that it takes patients for granted. Remember, patients' loyalties to their physicians are growing thinner than ever thanks to frequent changes in insurance plans, employers and residences. They don't need any help from your staff!

Registration workstation requirements

❑ Practice management system terminal

❑ All necessary forms

❑ Telephone

❑ Desktop photocopier or scanner

❑ Daily schedule (manual or automated)

❑ Office supplies

❑ Communication tool for patient arrival

Do your front office staff have to walk more than 10 feet to get to the nearest printer, photocopier or scanner? If so, the few extra seconds those additional footsteps take can add up to hours over the course of the year – time that would be better spent gathering and updating patient information, greeting incoming patients and seeing to other critical front desk tasks. Make sure your workstation is just that, a workstation with all of the resources needed by the front office staff. For more information on efficient workstations, see Chapter 2, "The Physician's Time."

 ...check-in procedures need improvement when you see...

- Front desk employees leaving the reception area for several minutes at a time to go into a separate room to photocopy insurance cards and do other registration tasks.

- Employees sitting at the front desk eating snacks while on break.

- A "take-a-number" system for registration.

- The sign-in sheet is on a ledge outside a closed sliding window with a sign on the window saying, "Knock if you need help."

- The triage nurse at the front desk talking to a patient on the telephone about a medical problem and doing so within earshot of the patients.

- Several $10 bills lying on top of the front office ledge.

- Urine samples sitting on the front office ledge for pickup.

The list of poor check-in practices witnessed in medical group practices, large and small, new and established, could go on for many pages. Let's just say there is room for improvement in all practices.

Do your front desk staff handwrite patient information changes for someone else to enter into the management system database later on? If so, you are just piling more work on your back office. In doing so, you are slowing cash flow by delaying charge entry and claims submission tasks. Real-time work processing is more efficient than batching work.

Now let's look at the various processes within the check-in function and see how each one works to support the entire function.

Take another view of registration

Complete accuracy in registration and pre-registration will save you much time and effort later on. But, no matter how you design your registration process, it must be patient-friendly. Too many medical practices have designed processes that may be practice-friendly or physician-friendly, but is definitely not patient-friendly.

Problems with claim rejections in your billing office?

- Study your front office processes and procedures. One internal medicine practice discovered that 10 percent of its claim rejections were direct results of registration problems – from ineligibility to incorrect policy numbers. In order to understand your registration errors, your billing staff must post rejections according to specific adjustment codes that can be reported on a summary basis. If you can't get information from your practice management system, take a sample of 500 claims and count the number of rejections by category versus the total number of claims.

- A multisite primary care practice found that reporting "the error rates" (the percent of claims rejected due to registration errors) to each of their 15 registration desks (one per site) on a weekly basis brought the point home...and the errors down. As your error rate decreases, the cost of billing declines, cash flow increases, and your staff work on the rejections generated by the insurance company, not their fellow staff members.

Pre-registration

Pre-registration is a process primarily used for new patients. However, some steps in the process are useful for gathering information from returning patients who may have changed insurance companies, addresses, telephone numbers, employers, or may have other important information changes. Any of these changes may affect what your staff must do to handle that patient's records, billing, financial responsibility, referral(s), prescription(s), and so forth.

Unless they have just walked in off the street unannounced, new patients will already have been in contact with someone on your staff, often through a telephone call to schedule the first appointment. If it is a referred patient, the initial contact to schedule the first appointment may have been with another physician's practice. Make the best of these contacts, however brief. They are your chance to gather some necessary information before the patient shows up for the appointment.

How much information is reasonable to gather from a referring practice when it makes an appointment for a new patient? Generally, you should be able to very quickly obtain the patient's name, home and work (and possibly cell) telephone numbers, the chief complaint, the insurance company and a referral number if the insurance company requires it. Or better yet, have the practice fax a registration form or face sheet for that patient.

Register patients when they call for appointments

The person who schedules appointments can either conduct a "mini registration" (gathering critical demographic and insurance information) or a "full registration" (all information needed for registration) at the same time the appointment is made.

This allows you to gather information in a timely manner. But some patients may not have all the information you need handy when they call. Your scheduling staff will also spend more time on the telephone with each patient, especially new ones. Smaller practices, where staff handle duties in several areas, may find this arrangement inflexible.

Recalling the commitment to real-time work processing, this registration process is the most efficient (until technology allows you to do it seamlessly). Since accuracy is more important – because it means that your practice will get paid – you may need to sacrifice real-time processing for accuracy and substitute an alternate form of registration as discussed below.

Transfer patients to a "pre-registration unit"

Immediately after the appointment is scheduled – but before patients hang up – transfer them to a specially staffed "pre-registration unit." Staff dedicated to this function can efficiently complete a mini- or full registration over the telephone.

Five ways to pre-register a patient (and their pluses and minuses)

❑ Register patients at the time they call for an appointment.

PLUS: Information is obtained in a timely manner.

MINUS: Patients may not have all needed information handy.
Staff spends more time on telephone and is unavailable for other duties.

❑ Transfer patients to a "pre-registration unit" immediately after they schedule.

PLUS: Makes the pre-registration process more efficient.

MINUS: The practice must have sufficient staff and telephone system.
Patients will hang up if forced to wait on hold for a long time and, if so, less information is gathered.

❑ Call patients back.

PLUS: Allows the practice to control the workflow of callbacks.

MINUS: May be difficult to track down patients.
Patients may view callbacks as inconvenient.

❑ Register patients over the Internet or via an Interactive Voice Response (IVR) system.

> **PLUS:** Convenient for patients and practice.

> **MINUS:** Patients may not complete all the necessary information.
> Not accessible to all patients.
> Technical glitches can happen.
> May raise security of information/privacy concerns (consult with your attorney).

❑ Register patients at a "pre-registration station" at your practice.

> **PLUS:** Keeps registration separate from "check-in" desk so fewer employees need to be specially trained and accountable for registration duties.

> **MINUS:** Patients often arrive at the clinical area and must be directed back to the "pre-registration unit." In a larger facility, that unit might even be on another floor. Unless you are mindful to request early arrival, new patients will arrive at their appointment time, not realizing that the "pre-registration unit" might consume up to 20 minutes and delay their actual appointment – and the productivity of your physicians.

This can make the entire pre-registration process much more efficient but you must have enough staff to pull it off. Call volumes can be unpredictable.

Don't get caught putting patients on hold for more than 15 seconds while they are transferred. Patients will feel inconvenienced and may hang up while on hold before your "pre-registration" information is gathered. Customer service should be an important consideration before embarking on this path, as your customers in the pre-registration process are largely new patients. Their first impression is an important one, and you don't want it to be that dealing with this practice always means an indefinite wait on hold.

Call patients back to complete pre-registration over the telephone

If the "pre-registration unit" is unavailable at the time the appointment is scheduled or the practice cannot dedicate sufficient staff to this function, the scheduler can gather some quick necessary information (insurance coverage and patient demographics). Then, the designated pre-registration staff can call the patient back later to do a full registration over the telephone.

Be prepared to play a little telephone tag: many patients won't be there when you attempt your call. Moreover, patients may find it intrusive if you call them back in the evening, even though that's when you have a better chance of contacting them.

Use better technology to pre-register patients

A sophisticated telephone system equipped with interactive voice response (IVR) software can capture registration information. The IVR software prompts patients who call into the system to provide all of the necessary registration information and records. Many patients adapt to this system quickly and find it easier than having to push buttons on their telephone keypads. The software communicates the patient's information to the practice's registration staff who then proceed with other registration tasks, such as insurance verification. IVR frees up staff time and, because staff can query and organize the database, it speeds many other registration functions. For example, you can quickly find all of the patients covered by a specific insurance plan and contact their insurance company for eligibility verification instead of going through all of the day's registration records one-by-one.

Insurance verification can ensure payment

Many insurance companies will give you access to their database of enrollees to help you verify that their beneficiary – and your patient – is actually covered by the insurance company they are claiming.

Gathering insurance information from your patients is important, but it cannot guarantee accuracy. Insurance cards are rarely stamped with the eligibility expiration date, and patients may abuse this fact or mistakenly provide you with inaccurate information. Insurance verification from the insurance company itself ensures that the patient is covered. (Although insurance companies update their systems often, please note that there may be terminations that have not yet been updated on their verification system. Although verification isn't a guarantee that the claim will be paid by the insurance company, it's the best tool that exists.)

On-line insurance verification can be done directly with the insurer or through a third-party vendor. On-line verification could occur during the interim between the time the patient schedules an appointment and the date of the appointment. This helps avoid the cost of dedicating more staff resources to calling insurers (and spending lots of time on hold). It also helps prevent claim denials that occur because the patient provided inaccurate coverage information or was not actually covered for the service your physicians provided.

If online access is unavailable, then the telephone is your next best option. Even though telephone verification may be more time-consuming for staff, the cost of denied or delayed claims is a much greater expense to the practice in the long run.

Don't limit your activities to verifying insurance coverage; determining the patient's eligibility for benefits is equally important. That is, if you are proceeding with infertility services on a patient covered by ABC Insurance, you'll want to make sure that the patient's contract with ABC Insurance covers infertility services. Determining benefits eligibility is particularly important for services that are not routinely covered by all insurance companies. Often, these are expensive services. Many insurance companies will provide the details of the patient's plan, including covered benefits, through online verification.

While you're at it, gather information about payments, including deductibles, copayments and coinsurance. Since these amounts can change often, patients are sometimes unaware of the most current obligations of their own insurance.

Finally, find out about covered laboratory and imaging facilities, referral and authorization requirements, as well as any other information that you can learn about the patient's plan that would help your practice.

Many practices have developed insurance verification and benefits eligibility forms that are completed and maintained for every patient.

The more data that you have prior to the patient's appointment, the better you can serve the patient and support the physician, and the greater the chances are that you will be paid appropriately for the services.

If you have limited resources for verification, consider limiting your verification activities to new patients, patients who are scheduled for procedures, surgeries or any other services that have fees in excess of $100 to $200 (that is, above the level of your "routine" services), and patients presenting to receive services that insurance companies may not cover (immunizations, nurse visits, etc.).

For surgical practices, this verification process should auto-matically be conducted for any patients scheduled for surgery at the time you call the insurance company for pre-authorization. The insurance company will inform you at that time if the patient is not on its roster. Thus, you could limit insurance verification activities to just those insurers that do not require pre-authorizations.

Don't make the pre-registration process unbearable to patients. If you decide to transfer callers to a pre-registration unit, the best way to create a dissatisfied patient is to put them on hold! Whatever method you choose for registration, make sure it provides top-notch customer service.

Although the pre-registration process itself is optional, collecting the information is not. Doing as much of it as possible before patients walk in the door will make their flow through the practice smoother and reduce administrative burdens on front and back office staff.

Registering patients via the Internet

Patients and staff alike will find Internet registration extremely convenient. Consider your patient population's ability to access the Internet before going down this road but, if you do, here are some tips to follow when giving your patients options to pre-register or update their information over the Internet.

✓ Electronic forms must be simple to complete and easy to submit. Patients accessing your Web site must be able to quickly find the forms on the site.

✓ Everything must work – no missing links, dead ends, etc.

✓ Use an experienced Internet provider.

✓ Make sure information can be easily loaded into your practice management information system; re-keying is a waste of time.

✓ Send patients a confirmation via e-mail that their information was received.

✓ Maintain a "print the form" option for those patients who are more comfortable completing forms by hand and bringing them to the practice for their appointment.

✓ Privacy is paramount. Discuss encryption and security options with your Internet provider. Make sure that your system meets HIPAA standards.

✓ If real-time data interchange is not available, ensure that patients are informed about when they should register prior to their appointments.

✓ Make sure that your online registration process works flawlessly with all of the most popular Internet browsers currently in use, including older versions.

✓ Try to make your online registration process as simple and straightforward as the ordering forms used on any major retailer's Web site; otherwise your attempts to increase convenience will be seen as incompetent.

Registration

Some parts of the check-in and registration processes cannot be done over the telephone, by mail, e-mail or otherwise. You will probably want the patient present to sign certain forms and confirm – just one more time – key information such as: current insurance company, address and telephone number(s). Face-to-face is also the best time to make sure that the patient has read and understands your practice's financial policy.

Greeting the patient

Do whatever you must in arranging workspace and job assignments but make sure that somebody actually greets patients as they enter the practice. Even if you do not make any of the egregious oversights of common sense and courtesy already listed in this chapter, you are still dropping the ball if your front desk staff:

- must also answer the bulk of incoming telephone calls while trying to deal face to face with patients;

- wear telephone headsets but make no effort to let patients know if they are talking to them or to someone on the telephone;

- have to constantly get up and search for the proper forms and for patient records; and/or

- do not have all the information they need to accurately answer or quick access to patients' most common questions such as the physician's timing (that is, running on schedule or not?) and billing questions.

...your registration process isn't working when you see staff walking around.

Do a mini time and motion study of the check-in process. How often does your front office staff have to get up and walk to a printer, copier or computer terminal? Multiply those extra seconds by the number of patients you register during a typical month. Now imagine what other tasks could have been attended to in that time.

Making staff walk just an extra 10 feet for each patient lengthens processing time, removes the employee from the greeting position, and tires the employee unnecessarily. Give your receptionists the tools needed to do the job at their workstations.

On-site registration of new patients

As with pre-registration, the on-site registration of new patients and established patients will require different administrative steps, information and time on your part.

If the patient has been pre-registered in one of the ways I've discussed, your staff must still verify that the information gathered so far is correct.

For new patients who have not pre-registered, your front office employees should have on hand a registration form that requests patients' demographic and insurance information. The form should also include the information presented under the section below on "necessary signatures," which will need to be presented to all new patients, regardless of whether they have been pre-registered.

Finally, collect the new patient's insurance card and, if considered helpful by the billing office, driver's license. Copy the cards on the photocopier or scan them on the scanner you have conveniently placed in the check-in area.

For optimum efficiency, set up the registration desk so staff can enter patient information directly into the practice's data system as soon as it is gathered from the patient. If, however, this direct keying cannot be done with accuracy, then simply gather the information and deliver it to a person(s) who can concentrate and key the information without error.

Asking to copy the patient's identification

THINGS TO CONSIDER

Make sure staff know that patients can refuse to allow photocopies of their drivers' licenses. Ask, "May we make a copy of your driver's license?"

If insurance verification has not been conducted, consider the process at this juncture. On-line or modem access is your best bet.

It used to be okay to photocopy or scan patients' insurance cards only once a year, but the labor market often dictates multiple employment changes, even within the year. It's time-consuming, but making a record of the card upon each visit or at least every three months improves your practice's odds of getting paid.

On-site registration of established patients

Be sure to ask established patients at registration if any of their key information has changed since they were last in. Do not assume that asking, "Has any information changed?" will bring the required response. Instead, ask a few specific questions, such as:

"Are you still located at 123 Anywhere Drive in Anyplace?"

"Do you still hold Anybody's Insurance?"

"Is your home telephone number still 555-1212?"

As with new patients, you should strive for optimum efficiency by recording any changes into your system on the spot. Real-time work processing is more efficient than batching work.

Cluttered Signage

I recently visited a practice where the reception room looked like a used car lot. Signs covered every spare ledge and nearly obscured the view into the registration area. The practice had posted notices about everything from its privacy policy to its expectations for time-of-service collections. The sheer volume of signage was bad enough, but the wording – the technical and legal jargon – on the signs was even worse.

Registration forms

Registration forms can be overwhelming to patients. It's easy to forget that most patients don't understand our insider abbreviations and regulatory lingo.

For all new patients and often for many of your established patients, you will develop and distribute a packet of information upon registration that includes your practice's forms, policies, procedures, and so forth. Although each practice will have its own set of forms, it's important for the information to be communicated clearly.

Here are some ways to make sure you communicate more effectively:

Keep words to seven letters. The average U.S. citizen reads at an elementary school level. Think about how many 10-letter words you knew in fourth grade; you could probably count them on one hand. Look for words with more than seven letters in your registration packet – "deductible," "nonparticipating," "compliant," "assignment of benefits." Is there a simpler word or phrase that you could substitute? Is there a simple explanation that you could give of the term?

Watch the abbreviations and acronyms. ABN, EOB, CMS – these mean nothing to many people. Take "HIPAA," for example. Do *you* know what the acronym stands for? Even many health industry gurus get confused about it. Your patients will, too, if you hand them a complex Notice of Privacy Practices form and simply say, "HIPAA requires it." If you use the terms, explain them.

Take your registration packet home. Ask your spouse, neighbor, or even your 12-year-old to look at it. If they can't understand it (assuming they don't work in health care), your patients won't either.

Unless you have an EMR, **consider color-coding your forms.** Your registration forms could be light green, for example, contrasting with yellow phone message and lab results forms, blue health history forms and white office notes.

Understand regulatory requirements; don't just pass them along. For example, the "Notice of Privacy Practices" required by HIPAA. Some practices use a complex template that was drafted by a lawyer and is more than seven pages long. Some legal language is required, of course, but take time to understand what HIPAA requires you to include in the privacy notice and figure out how to say it simply. For example: "We will call you to remind you about appointments" makes much more sense than "Expect telephonic, minimum-necessary communication concerning upcoming opportunities for compliance."

Provide scripts and educate your front desk staff. It is much more efficient for staff at the front desk to answer patients' questions about ABNs, HIPAA, time-of-service payments, medical records release and so forth. Teach your staff what various forms are used for and provide them with lists of frequently asked questions and the appropriate answers.

Simplicity is key when communicating to patients about regulations, policies, money owed or, really, anything else. Patients aren't stupid; they just don't live and breathe our health care jargon.

Necessary signatures

In order to seek payment from insurance companies on behalf of your patients for services rendered, there are several agreements to which patients must attest. They do this by reading and indicating by signature that they understand those agreements. Many of these agreements are signed one-time only when they register as new patients. Others must be renewed at each visit.

The most common agreements for which you seek the patient's signature are provided below; however, be sure to review them carefully for appropriate use in your practice.

Assignment of Benefits: The patient agrees to assign his or her insurance benefits to the practice so the practice may bill and receive payment on his or her behalf. Form should be signed by every new patient and upon change of insurance.

Form C-1
Assignment of Benefits

I hereby assign to XYZ Practice any insurance or other third-party benefits available for health care services provided to me. I understand that XYZ Practice has the right to refuse or accept assignment of such benefits. If these benefits are not assigned to XYZ Practice, I agree to forward to XYZ Practice all health insurance and other third-party payments that I receive for services rendered to me immediately upon receipt.

_____

Signature of Patient/Legal Guardian   Date_____

Medical Records Release: The patient agrees to permit the practice to release medical records on his behalf to third parties. This includes medical documentation requested by insurance companies when a claim is disputed. The form should be signed by new patients and upon change of insurance.

Form C-2
Authorization for Release of Information

I authorize XYZ Practice to release all medical information (including, but not limited to, information on psychiatric conditions, sickle cell anemia, alcohol and drug abuse, and HIV or communicable diseases) requested by my health insurance company, Medicare or any other third-party payers. I authorize XYZ Practice to release all medical information to my referring physician and my primary (family) physician. I authorize XYZ Practice to contact my insurance company or health plan administrator and obtain all pertinent financial information concerning coverage and payments under my policy. I direct the insurance company or health plan administrator to release such information to XYZ Practice. I agree that these provisions

---

will remain in effect until I provide written revocation to XYZ Practice.

_____
Signature of Patient/Legal Guardian Date_____

Waiver Form: The patient agrees to be responsible for service(s) that the practice recognizes the insurance company will not pay. One form – Insurance Coverage Waiver – should be used for patients for whom insurance coverage cannot be verified. Another form – Non-Covered Services – should be used for specific services that an insurance company will not cover. These waiver forms should be signed only when circumstances dictate. The non-covered services form should be used only for services that the physician knows will not be covered by insurance.

Form C-3
Insurance Coverage Waiver
    I understand that my eligibility for coverage by (name of insurance company) cannot be confirmed at this time. I wish to receive medical service from (name of physician). If it is determined that I am not eligible for coverage, I understand that I will be responsible for payment of all services provided.

_____
Signature of Patient/Legal Guardian Date_____

Form C-4
Non-Covered Services*

Your insurance company will only pay for services that it determines to be medically necessary. If your insurance company determines that a particular service, although it would otherwise be covered, is not medically necessary, your insurance company will deny payment for that service. I believe that, in your case, your insurance company is likely to deny payment for one or more of the following reasons: [Statement regarding the service being provided and why the insurancecompany is likely to deny payment.]

I have been notified by my physician that he/she believes that, in my case, my insurance company is likely to deny payment for the service identified above, for the reasons stated. If my insurance company denies payment, I agree to be personally and fully responsible for payment.

_____
Signature of Patient/Legal Guardian Date _____

*Please note that you'll need to make sure that the insurance company does not have a specific policy to which you agreed in your contract with them **prohibiting** you from collecting payment from patients for non-covered services.*

Financial Policy: This optional, but highly recommended, form briefly states in non-legalese the practice's billing and payment policies. The patient's signature indicates that he or she understands and agrees to the practice's financial policies. Signature is required according to practice's policy; it should be signed by new patients and each time a patient changes insurance coverage.

Form C-5
Components of a Financial Policy

- Why your policy is in writing.

- Why you need to update personal information each visit (or based on your practice's policy).

- What payment is required at the time of service.

- The allowable forms of payment.

- Your collections cycle.

- Who patients can contact in the practice if they have any questions.

- The role of your collections agency.

- Statement regarding the responsibility of a patient for the total charge.

- Statement regarding the practice's policy on insurance assignment.

- Statement regarding the practice's collection system (including interest charges or other fees, if applicable).

Advance Beneficiary Notice (ABN): An ABN is a written notification made to a Medicare beneficiary before items or services are furnished for which the physician believes that Medicare will decline to reimburse. Although an ABN is included in this "Registration" section, it is likely that clinical staff will use this form at the point of care when the service is provided, rather than front desk staff. Find a detailed description of the ABN, when it is needed and the required forms at www.cms.gov.

Notice of Privacy Release: The privacy regulations of the Health Insurance Portability and Accountability Act (HIPAA) require physicians who have a direct treatment relationship with an individual to post a notice of privacy practices in a "clear and permanent position" in the office. In addition to posting the notice, patients must acknowledge the notice by signing or initialing a copy. This is not a consent form, rather it is an acknowledgement. Find a sample form at www.physicianspractice.com.

Make your staff part of continuous registration improvement

(WISDOM)

■ Consider the registration process an integral function of your billing operation.

■ Involve registration staff in billing meetings and written communications about billing practices.

■ Base part of employee performance measurements on registration error rates because accurate registration information will positively affect your practice's cash flow. Obtain this information from edit reports from your electronic claims transmission and/or the denial codes printed on the explanation of benefits (EOBs).

■ Make sure new staff training for registration personnel includes a two to three week rotation in the billing office so they can understand their integral role in the billing process.

■ Create a registration "certification" process. All staff members who register patients must pass a proficiency test to ensure that they are qualified. Don't limit this process to new employees; ensure proficiency annually for all staff who register patients.

■ Count over a 30-day period the number of claims that come back and need rework because some piece of patient information was not gathered or updated at registration. You may be amazed. Share this information with staff.

Steps to Get You There: Follow the Paperwork Reduction Plan

Many physicians ask new patients to bring in all of their medications for a thorough review. Why not conduct a similar review of your practice's paperwork? Gather up the forms you ask your patients to sign. Spread the forms out on a table. As you do, look for:

1. **Forms you don't need.** One hospital-owned practice still used a form that the chief financial officer had insisted on five years earlier. The form was no longer needed. Throwing it out cut 90 seconds off of each patient's registration. Ninety seconds per patient adds up to a lot of staff time by the end of the month. Another practice handed out a separate form describing its $25 charge for no-shows. Yet, the practice had never charged a no-show patient and had no intention of doing so. Solution? Toss the form.

2. **Forms that could be combined.** Administrative goals and clinical staff must find common ground. Gathering information in one thorough process instead of several different ones saves money and time.

3. **Forms that contain misinformation or mistakes.** Look for misspelled words and requirements that are no longer applicable.

4. **Forms that are ugly or illegible.** You can only photocopy a form so many times before it becomes difficult to read. Worse, it makes your practice look amateur, which is not a good way to build patients' confidence.

Be critical, but don't go overboard. If you eliminate essential forms, required information or forms that could save the physician time in the exam room, you'll soon be adding more forms.

Sometimes you can't make everybody happy

One physician wanted each patient's name in the top right-hand corner of the registration form. Another wanted it in the top left-hand corner. Accommodating such divergent requests is arguably manageable in a two-physician practice, but it would be next to impossible to try and satisfy the preferences of 55 different physicians – and still run an efficient practice. Physicians who understand the group practice concept know that many times administrative policies must be based on what is best for the group, which is not always the same as what each individual wishes.

The sign-in list

Think about it, a major compromise to patient privacy and a leading source of discourtesy to patients is probably sitting almost right under your nose! It is the ubiquitous sign-in list. These lists compromise patient confidentiality because they display for all the world to see every preceding patient's name, appointment time, physician's name and other information, such as insurance company, home telephone number, and so on.

Once upon a time, the sign-in list was used primarily to gauge the patient's arrival time. It gave staff a way to manage the time it took to process patients who arrived at irregular and unpredictable times.

Unfortunately, in too many practices, this list has evolved to replace the function of greeting patients. How many times have I seen an employee seated at a registration desk tell a patient to "sign in" without even looking up and acknowledging the individual? More than I can count. Then, in all too many practices, the patient is ignored until called back up to the front desk to register. Even worse is posting a sign telling patients to sign in, then ignoring them for the next 15 minutes.

Greet and acknowledge patients as they arrive. Eliminate the sign-in list, particularly on slow days. It will force your front office to process work on a real-time basis.

HIPAA does not require you to eliminate patient sign-in sheets. You can still use sign-in sheets and comply with HIPAA. That said, limit what you ask patients to write on this form to the minimum amount of information necessary to identify that the patient has arrived for his scheduled visit.

Do a better job of handling the sign-in part of the check-in function, and your practice will go a long way toward improving patient relations and operating its patient flow more efficiently.

Make the check-in process work in your favor

1. **Greet your patients.** Say, "Hi, how are you doing today?" instead of immediately directing them to the sign-in list and barely acknowledging their presence.

2. **"Hire" a volunteer greeter.** Call your local senior citizen's center and ask for volunteer greeters.

3. **Eliminate the sign-in list.** Real-time registration is a much more efficient way to process patients.

4. **Use a sign-in "label" or "pad" system.** Ask patients to write vital sign-in information on an individual piece of paper. Then, place the labels or notes in the order of arrival (or pre-printed with numbers) on a list kept at the front desk (but out of the patients' view).

Communicating the patient's arrival

The patient has registered and signed in. Now, you have to let clinical staff – who are often in another part of the office – know that the patient has arrived and is ready for the appointment.

Here are some of the most common methods of communicating the patient's arrival:

Line of Sight: Once the patient is processed, place the chart where those at the nurses' station can see it. A chart rack can be placed on a ledge, counter or wall. A strategically positioned mirror (convex or flat depending on the space) can create a line of sight if necessary.

Lighting System: Lights can be used to indicate a patient's arrival. Someone at the reception desk can press a switch that turns on a lamp bulb at the nurses' station. Practices with more than one provider can use lights of different colors or flashing patterns. However, this type of system may not work well in a practice where nurses or other back office staff are away from their stations frequently. For a large office, consider installing a lighting system outside and inside of each exam room, as well as at the nurses' station.

Buzzers or Chimes: These work through the telephone system or a separate low voltage system. Caution: buzzers or chimes that are too loud or have an irritating tone will quickly wear out their welcome with the people who have to listen to them day after day. These may not be useful if the nurses are all in the exam rooms.

Charge Ticket Print Out: Place a printer in (or adjacent to) the nurses' station. When a patient has arrived and is ready to be seen, the reception desk staff prints out the patient's charge ticket on that printer. This helps maintain the chart in the nurses' station, allowing the clinical team to review it prior to the patient's arrival. It also helps to ensure accuracy for staff who rely on the charge ticket's registration information for making referrals, scheduling procedures and so on.

Pagers or Radios: Give the clinical staff pagers that can print out text messages (e.g., the patient's last name, first initial). Registration staff can call the pager when a patient is ready. In this arrangement, the clinical assistant who retrieves the patient can easily retrieve charts from the front office. Alternately, the charts can be kept in the nurses' station. Two-way radios can play a similar role, but with voice transactions instead of text messaging. Be aware that information broadcast on a radio or intercom might be audible to other patients so keep comments brief and pay attention patient confidentiality if you use them.

Messaging Systems: As with pagers, messaging systems, such as internal e-mail, instant messaging or OmniNote®, can be used to transmit the arrival information, but in more detail.

Digital Wireless Phones: Use portable wireless telephones that integrate with your existing telephone system. This option allows your front office to call or send text messages via wireless phones to clinical assistants wherever they are in the practice.

Practice Management System: In some systems, the scheduling module allows users to indicate the patient's "arrival" once registration is completed. If your system offers this feature, place a terminal in the nurses' station or suspend the monitor from a wall or ceiling. Remember to keep the screen out of patients' sight for confidentiality reasons.

Although a messaging system can facilitate the communication of the patients' arrival, it shouldn't be the only bridge between the "front" and the "back." In order to work as a team, your practice needs these employees to be in constant communication.

Don't let registration and check-in snafus disrupt the patient flow process. You can handle the registration and check-in steps more efficiently and effectively with the right tools, right processes and a well-trained staff.

"Mr. Smith, front and center!"

Did you ever consider that a clinical assistant poking his head into the reception area and yelling out a name might not be the best way to retrieve patients? Instead, try one of these ideas to make this process friendlier:

1. Take photographs of new patients (with their permission, of course), and attach the photos to their charts or store the digital image in the patients' electronic medical records to help staff find patients in the reception area.

2. Photocopy patients' driver's licenses (after asking for permission, of course) and secure copies to charts to help staff identify patients in the reception area.

3. Instruct the receptionist to write down a brief description of what patients are wearing (but nothing that you would be embarrassed for patients to see).

4. When new patients register, ask how they would like to be addressed. Note their response prominently in the chart so you can at least refer to patients in their preferred manner when you do have to communicate with them.

Exam room registration

If you have been unlucky enough to be an emergency room walk-in patient lately, you may have noticed that you didn't have to stop by the ER's front office. They came to you. Why? "Bedside registration" is all the rage in emergency rooms because it streamlines the check-in process, eliminates patient waiting time and makes better use of staff time.

Can this streamlined approach work in a medical practice? You bet. The concept is catching on in medical practices, and it's working extraordinarily well at reducing cycle time. (See Chapter 6, "Waiting Room," for more information on cycle time.)

Exam room registration can eliminate some of your front office processes, as well as most of the space that you have to allocate for the front office and the waiting room. Staffing reductions are also possible because it allows you to combine front office staff and clinical assistant positions into a new staff position called the patient service representative (PSR).

How does it work? PSRs escort patients directly into the exam room to conduct the registration process as soon as they arrive. Depending on the volume, a greeter can be stationed near the doorway in which patients enter the practice to direct them back to the exam room area where the PSRs would be waiting, or to communicate to the PSRs (through a wireless phone, for example) that a patient has arrived and is ready to be escorted back.

After the patient is escorted or directed into the exam room, your PSR staff can register patients, collect payments, take vital signs, help patients fill out medical histories and perform other rooming duties.

In other words, your patient will have only one stop (the exam room), instead of two (the waiting room and the exam room), and one staff (the PSR), instead of two (the receptionist and the clinical assistant).

To ease the transition to this model without major remodeling or staff disruptions, hire medical assistants as your front office staff turns over. Alternately, you can train nonmedical front-office employees who show the potential for the new position of patient service representative.

Escorting patients directly to their exam room avoids shuffling patients from one waiting area – the waiting room – to another waiting area, which is what exam rooms become when you use them to park patients. Forcing patients to wait in several locations seems to increase the perceived amount of time they spend waiting for a physician.

The arrangement only works well if the process of clinical intake does not require a nurse. That said, many physicians repeat their nurse's duties anyway. That is, when the physician walks into the exam room after the patient has been processed, she re-takes the patient's medical history, re-reviews all medications, re-reviews the complaint from the very first symptom and so forth. While many physicians want to reconfirm this information, the physician who routinely ignores all of the information gathered by the nurse — or does not trust that information — gains little efficiency from the current intake process and may transition well into this new model of exam room registration.

Exam room registration also requires a robust pre-visit process in which insurance verification and benefits eligibility are conducted *before* the patient arrives. Find out more about pre-registration functions elsewhere in this chapter. Although there are significant efficiencies to be gained through the model, you wouldn't want to lose revenue because of errors in your billing process by switching.

Depending on the size, specialty and volume of patients at your practice, you might want to use two patient service representatives for each physician or three PSRs for every two physicians. You might also ask a nurse to oversee and supplement these care teams.

Exam room registration is particularly valuable for practices that serve a patient population that does not speak English or in which many patients speak English as a second language. The care teams for these practices can include staff who speak your patient panel's primary languages other than English. For example, if Spanish and Russian are the primary languages for sufficient numbers of your patients, then include a Spanish-speaking PSR and a Russian-speaking PSR on each team. The PSRs also can interpret for the physicians and other clinical staff by remaining in the exam room with the caregiver even after the registration and intake process are complete.

A few practices go so far as to build facilities with exam room doors that open directly to the parking lot. Patients enter exam rooms where customer service representatives meet them and perform the registration and intake process. Your practice may not be ready for that step yet but using the process in your present facility will definitely speed patient registration and soothe patient frustrations.

However you implement it, to make exam room registration work, your practice must collapse its two check-in processes — the administrative and the clinical — into one process.

This is the main benefit of exam room registration: it allows you to combine clinical and administrative functions to save space, time and staff costs.

Chapter 6

WAITING

Key Chapter Lessons

> Analyze your waiting times

> Evaluate your cycle time

> Learn ways to occupy your patients as they wait

> Identify options to reduce waiting times

> Recognize the value of communicating to your staff and your patients

Advanced Concepts

> Calculate wait time

The waiting process

We have built our medical practices around the concept that patients will wait for us. In fact, we even dare to call it a "waiting room!" With that mindset, it's no wonder that abuses abound at this step in the patient flow process. It should be no secret that improvements in communications and increasing expectations are making people less "patient" than ever.

Do you know your practice's average wait time?

Surveys by the American Medical Association indicate that the average time patients spend in the physician's waiting room is 19 minutes. Waiting times vary from specialty to specialty. If your average wait time is more than 20 minutes, what extra efforts are you taking to entertain patients while they wait? Even if less than 20 minutes, is your practice's wait time longer than the average for the specialty of your physicians? Do you know your practice's average wait time by day, by week and by month – so you can intervene with changes to operating systems and procedures to bring this to acceptable levels?

Cycle Time

Cycle time is the measurement of time from the patient's entry to the patient's exit. The cycle time in a medical practice, typically from 30 to 90 minutes, can be divided into process time (value-added) and wait time (non-value-added). Process time includes the actual time of registration, the actual time of the provision of care, the actual time of checkout; wait time is all of the time spent waiting between or during processes.

Patients can help you measure cycle time

If you don't have time to conduct your own timing survey to analyze wait time, let your patients do the study for you. Give every patient a clipboard with a survey instrument that highlights each point at which the patient should record the time (for example, check-in, escort to the back, etc.). Be forewarned that patients' perceptions will influence the survey, and do not try this if waiting is a significant problem in your practice. You may infuriate your patients by asking them to measure the waiting that they dread!

Cycle time

What is your practice's cycle time? In an efficient medical practice, cycle time – how long it takes a patient to get in and out of the door – averages less than 60 minutes. Of course, procedures, many ancillaries and complicated office visits will take longer.

Unfortunately, most practices seem reconciled to a long patient cycle time. Many practices make things worse by escorting patients to exam rooms long before the physician is ready to see them. It doesn't reduce total waiting time at all. It doesn't fool the patient. And it can waste staff time. Nurses and medical assistants who are kept busy escorting patients to exam rooms have less time for patient work ups and the other tasks that maximize physicians' time with patents.

Many practices are focusing on cycle time to reduce patient waiting time. Here's how you can get started.

Measure cycle time. Start the clock when a patient enters your practice and stop the clock when he leaves. That's one cycle. Ask staff at the front desk to note the exact time that each patient signs in, assuming that patients don't have to wait in line to sign in. The checkout time can be noted at the conclusion of the checkout process.

Assess cycle time. Refine your cycle time assessment. Calculate the average cycle time for the patients whose visits make up 80 percent of your physician's typical office visits.

Target one area for improvement. Measure check-in time, for example. Can you make it go faster by reducing the amount of paperwork that patients must complete? Can you pre-register patients online or by phone? Reevaluate check-in time after making changes and assuring that the portions of the process you change are running smoothly.

Re-measure total cycle. After making changes in the area targeted for improvement, measure check-in time again, as well as the total cycle time for the average patient visit. Did cycle time go down, stay the same or go up? Be careful that you do not just transfer a time-consuming process from one area to another. Target another portion of the patient flow process for improvements and repeat the process.

There is no "perfect" cycle time, but maximizing value-added time (the actual encounter between the patient and the physician) and minimizing non-value added time (asking patient's insurance information for the fifth time) creates a win/win situation for you and your patients.

Try to strike a healthy balance so patients and physicians spend more time together and both spend less time waiting for each other.

Where to attack waiting time

1. **Eliminate check-in.** If your clinical intake process does not require a nurse, staff your front desk with patient service representatives who are trained to register and room patients, take vital signs, help patients fill out medical histories and other duties.

2. **Eliminate the waiting room.** If your practice can verify insurance and benefits eligibility before the patient arrives, conduct the registration process in the exam room. Emergency rooms do something similar, known as "bedside registration."

   (See Advanced Concept, "Exam Room Registration," in Chapter 5 for more information on eliminating check-in and the waiting room.)

3. **Eliminate checkout altogether.** Collect time-of-service payments upfront at check-in. Process any referrals, schedule tests and arrange any follow-up appointments in the exam room. Stop giving the patients charge tickets to carry to another desk – just let them go after the exam.

4. **Think out of the box.** Find a solution that works for your specialty and your practice. Imagine new possibilities, and you may surprise yourself – and your patients.

How to make the wait go faster

The nature of your practice's services, the fact that every patient is unique, and the fact that the exact arrival of your patients is unpredictable mean that you will never be able to achieve an average wait time of zero minutes in your practice. But there are many ways to make the waiting process more bearable.

Change your "waiting room" to a "reception area." Changing what you call that area where patients wait before their appointment can help to create a new attitude for staff and patients. Support this by changing signage, as well as how your staff refers to the area.

Add amenities. Your reception area and exam rooms should provide entertainment or at least occupy your patients as they wait. Offer refreshments such as water and coffee. Make sure magazines are current and books are of interest to your patient population and their family members. Play calming music and pay attention to lighting the room in such a way that it is relaxing but not dim.

A professional secret shopper's checklist

A professional secret shopper offers her "shopping" test for medical practices.

Front Office

- ☐ Did the receptionist smile?
- ☐ Were you greeted immediately upon approaching?
- ☐ Did the receptionist use eye contact?
- ☐ Did the receptionist ask if you needed help?
- ☐ Was the receptionist well-groomed and clean?
- ☐ Was a friendly attitude projected?
- ☐ Were you assisted in a timely manner?
- ☐ How long did you wait for someone to acknowledge you?
- ☐ If the receptionist was running late, were you informed of an approximate time you would be assisted?
- ☐ How long did you wait past your scheduled appointment?
- ☐ Did the receptionist acknowledge the delay with an apology or other acknowledgment?
- ☐ If the receptionist was unable to answer your question, did he or she seek out someone who could?
- ☐ Were all of your questions answered to your satisfaction?
- ☐ Were you thanked or invited to return?
- ☐ Was the associate knowledgeable about product or service?
- ☐ Was the telephone answered in three rings or less?

☐ Was the receptionist on the telephone courteous towards you?

Facility

☐ Was the outside of the building clean and free of debris?

☐ Was the entryway clean and well-maintained?

☐ Was the indoor temperature comfortable – not too warm or too cold?

☐ Were the restrooms clean, stocked and in good working order?

☐ Was the patient lobby comfortable and inviting?

☐ In the patient lobby, were the sick patients separated from the well patients?

☐ In the patient lobby, were the magazines current and well-maintained?

☐ Were the exam rooms clean and well-maintained?

☐ In the exam rooms, did patients have access to copies of health-related articles that are specific to patients' needs?

Source: Stacy Dunevitz, Professional Secret Shopper. Used with permission.

Reception area do's and a don't

■ Provide patients with notepads or coloring books for children with your logo.

■ Make your reception area informative by providing patients with literature about your practice and educational materials pertinent to your practice.

■ Offer a blank form with heading: "Things I wish to discuss with my doctor today." This allows patients to consider the information they want to convey to the physician so that the patient-physician interaction is more focused.

■ Use calming, but cheerful colors.

■ Don't fill your reception area with couches; most patients without family members will wish to sit by themselves.

Maintain the area. Children's toys should not be scattered about for someone to trip on. Torn or outdated magazines should be removed. Carpets should be clean. The walls should not be dirty or have significant marks on them. Trash should be picked up nightly, or even twice a day. Someone should be designated for the responsibility to walk through the area frequently throughout the day to tidy up.

Add other reception area amenities. Consider other ways to make the wait go faster for patients by adding some of the following amenities:

- Patient education materials.

- Internet connectivity or a PC loaded with the practice's Web site.

- Telephone with free local access.

- AccentHealth®(free health station and TV for physician offices).

- Jigsaw puzzles (but not for practices where there will be very small children who could choke on a small piece). Take a puzzle to a craft store to be mounted, have the patient who put the final piece in the puzzle sign it, and hang it as a decoration.

- A toy bin for children but, again, make sure toys are safe and are not left where other, especially older, patients could stumble on them and fall. Recognizing that toys should be cleaned after every play session by a child (to prevent infection), many practices now encourage parents to bring their child's own toy(s).

- Recipe and coupon exchange boxes.

- Pagers to allow patients to get up and walk around if there is a shopping area, mall or outdoor walking area adjacent to the practice.

- Community board with information about support groups, exercise activities, etc.

- Rotating "art gallery" of local artists' work. In addition to showcasing local talent, your reception area will be decorated — for free! Rotate the "show" every six months.

- Pictures of physicians, staff and their families with professional and personal information about their lives in order to establish a "personal" relationship between the patients and your practice. Try baby pictures as well – your patients will be delighted.

- Coloring page featuring an image of a physician and a patient and a couple of crayons or pens. Search for one of several Web sites that feature images of physicians with patients that can be printed for free. Insert your logo for instantaneous marketing; the coloring page will soon be hanging on many refrigerators in your community.

- Word scramble featuring content relevant to your specialty. Search for one of several Internet sites that allow you to create one for free.

Entertaining your patients won't eliminate the wait, but it will make it more tolerable.

The waiting room becomes a nicer place to wait

Harbour Health is a group of 18 health care providers specializing in family practice and obstetrics and gynecology. In addition to ancillary services, the group includes physicians, midwives, nurse practitioners, physician assistants, an acupuncturist, massage therapist, herbalist, lactation consultant and a nutritionist.

"Our waiting room is a large area with various groupings of furniture placed around the area, living room style. In the center, we have placed a glass table with a large silk floral arrangement. When patients enter the waiting room, they head to the reception desk where we have two staff members on duty. After they are checked in, patients are directed to the furniture grouping closest to the doorway that the medical assistant will use when she comes to get them. (There are three patient doorways into the clinical areas). In addition, on one side of the waiting room, the patient can access Path LAB (a private laboratory to whom we lease space) and our mammography services.

"Because our area has a strong community of artists and craftspeople, we rotate the artwork on our waiting room walls with 'shows' from local artists. At no cost to our organization, we have an ever-changing variety of exceptional artwork on display while performing a service to the artists.

"In each grouping of chairs and tables, we provide materials on various health issues or preventative health information, as well as current magazines. We have a large bulletin board in the waiting room that announces community events as well as promotes the classes and seminars we provide on a regular basis – to include a 'boot camp' for new fathers."

Patty Royer, Administrator, Harbour Health, Portsmouth, NH

Keep a pulse on your practice

Why wait for the results of your patient satisfaction survey? To keep a pulse on patient flow and the practice in general, the manager at an East Coast orthopedic practice walks through the reception area twice a day to talk to the patients. She says the 15 minutes she spends over the course of the day doing the walk-throughs are the most valuable minutes of her day!

Can you eliminate waiting?

The short answer is "no" — no matter how adept you are at scheduling patients, your average waiting time will never be reduced to zero. Unlike the efficiency of a manufacturing operation, providing a service is very susceptible to many factors, including variations in demand. For example, if every patient presented in 15-minute intervals (not even a minute off) and it took your office exactly 15 minutes to serve each one (again, not even a minute off), then you could create a no-waiting environment. But let's get real; we can neither expect every patient to present at exact intervals nor their service time to be exact. Don't forget that your service is perishable. That is, the "service" — your physicians' time — cannot be inventoried or stored until the patient arrives. So what are your options? You have three basic options:

Smooth demand through scheduling techniques. Encourage your patients to schedule their flu shots before the big rush comes by including a reminder note in your patient statements (see Chapter 4, "Scheduling" for more tips on managing patient demand).

Adjust service capacity. Use part-time physicians, flexible work shifts, and introduce patient co-production (see the Advanced Concept, "The Patient as Co-producer," in Chapter 7, "The Patient Encounter," for more information about co-production). Study your physician's schedule to ensure you have the proper level of staff to match the demands created by the schedule. If all of your physicians want the Monday morning clinic, hire additional front office staff to serve your patients on that morning. Don't forget to use idle capacity to your advantage; give the task of opening mail to your telephone operators, for example.

Allow customers to wait. Knowing that your patients will have to wait, at least, try to occupy their time to make the wait go faster. Does this mathematical fact mean that you should give up on minimizing wait times? No way! Managing your wait times to minimize them is important to patient satisfaction. A patient waiting four minutes to see the physician will be much happier than a patient who must wait 40, no matter how many jigsaw puzzles there are to pursue.

When being extra nice to patients is fraud

Waiving the copayment for patients who have endured lengthy waits may sound like a good idea, but if you do it consistently, be advised that insurance companies will consider it fraud. Why? Because waiving a copayment interferes with the contractual relationship between the employer, insurer and beneficiary. This waiver is no different than any other waiver. Waiving copayments on a routine basis is suspect on a number of grounds; routinely waiving copayments effectively reduces the practice's fee schedule. If you consistently reduce the patient's portion, insurance companies will expect the same courtesy; that is, they expect to be given a discount as well. However, you can still try to mend fences with patients who have put up with long waits by offering them a coupon for a discounted beverage at a nearby café or cafeteria. Just make sure that whatever you offer is of nominal cash value.

Other tips for the reception area

Communicate the wait time. When any staff member (nurse, medical assistant, receptionist, etc.) learns that a physician is unable to arrive on time or must cancel scheduled office hours, this information should be communicated immediately to all staff. Patients who are already waiting should be informed by the physician's clinical assistant and asked if they would prefer to wait (if it's an option) or be rescheduled. At the same time, the administrative staff (preferably an appointment scheduler) should contact the other patients affected by the physician's delay and reschedule them.

When the physician is running more than 30 minutes behind schedule, tell newly arriving patients of the delay. Keep currently waiting patients informed and offer to reschedule their appointments if they so choose. Be sure to have a contingency plan that identifies who is responsible for what so that responsibilities for the tasks of communicating, rescheduling and processing are clear.

Be fair to your staff. Don't let the front office bear the brunt of patients' frustrations over long waiting times. The idea of placing a sign in the reception area that says, "Please see the receptionist if you have been waiting longer than 20 minutes," can be unfair to staff when they must constantly apologize (and contend with angry patients) for a physician who consistently runs well behind schedule. Not informing the front office about an emergency surgery that delays the physician leaves a receptionist vulnerable to angry patients who become even more agitated when the receptionist admits no knowledge of what's going on.

Your physicians may believe that their patients are "willing to wait" but that is not always the case. Many patients actually have other things on their schedule besides a doctor's appointment. Give patients and staff the information that they need.

Recognizing that waiting is inevitable should foster creative solutions to keep your patients informed, occupied and, possibly, entertained. Although waiting will occur, this fact is not an excuse to tolerate long waits in your practice; don't let an entertaining reception area lull your practice into accepting hour-long waits. Instead, measure and monitor wait times, using ideas that you learn in this book to reduce waiting during and between processes.

ADVANCED CONCEPT

Calculating wait time

If you were presented with evidence that a function provided by your practice results in long waiting times for your patients, how would you troubleshoot the problem? How would you estimate the impact of changes in process versus changes in staffing to reduce long wait times? For example, can you determine how an increase in staff can reduce the wait time? A basic formula borrowed from industrial engineering (a field rich with methods for measuring and analyzing wait times in production and service processes) provides a quick, practical method. As demonstrated, this simple formula works to estimate average wait times and evaluate the relative impact of process versus staff changes.

Let's use the example of an in-house laboratory to demonstrate this concept:

1. Count the number of patient arrivals per hour (that is, how many patients seek out or are referred to the lab).

2. Determine the average lab processing time (that is, how long it takes on average for a technician to process a patient in the laboratory; include the time that the technician works with or on the patient and the test).

3. Count the number of technicians who staff the laboratory.

$W_b = 1 / (\mu - \lambda)$

Whereas m = average service rate per lab technician (defined as the average rate of patients processed per hour per technician);

λ = patient arrivals per technician; and

W_b = waiting time

Your lab is staffed by three technicians, who all handle the same services (i.e., there are not any tests that must be performed by any one technician; all are cross-trained). Twenty patients come to the lab each hour. The average processing time for each patient (preparation, drawing and holding) is six minutes; that is, each technician has the capacity to handle 10 patients per hour.

μ = 10 [average rate of 10 patients per hour per technician]

λ = 6.667 [20 arrivals per hour/3 technicians]

W_b = 1/ (10-6.667)

= 1/3.333

= .3 hours

= 18 minutes [.3 hours * 60 minutes]

Each of your patients will have to wait, on average, 18 minutes. Holding the volume of patients constant, if you want to bring the wait time down, either change the process (e.g., five-minute processing time would reduce the patient wait time to 11.3 minutes) or change the staffing (e.g., four full-time equivalent employees would reduce the wait time to 12 minutes). Of course, I'd recommend changing the process if at all possible, as adding staff will definitely add expenses, while process re-engineering may not.

Try measuring your average wait time for your registration staff using the same formula:

$W_b = 1 / (\mu - \lambda)$
Whereas μ = average service rate per registrar;

λ = patient arrivals per registrar; and
W_b = waiting time

Your registration desk is staffed by _____(a)_____ registrars, who all handle the same services (i.e., there are not any registration functions that must be performed by any one registrar; all are cross-trained). _____(b)_____ patients come to the registration desk each hour. The average processing time for each patient registration is _____(c)_____ minutes.

μ = 60 (minutes)/(c)
λ = (b)/(a)
$W_b = 1/(\mu - \lambda)$

Don't forget to divide by 60 to convert your result to minutes. You can do this test for the functions in your office in which employees perform identical functions. Because nurses, for example, perform different functions depending on the physician's request, you cannot run the same analysis for this staff function.

Note: Using the M/M/c model, this analysis assumes the demand for service times is assumed to be constant. That is, during the morning session, service begins at 9:00 a.m. and finishes at 5:00 p.m. with a steady flow of patients seeking lab services. For further information on waiting times, please see E.J. Rising, et al, "A Systems Analysis of a University Health-Service Outpatient Clinic," Operations Research, vol. 21, no. 5, Sept.-Oct. 1973; and J. Fitzsimmons and M. Fitzsimmons, Service Management, Chapters 11 and 17, 1998.

Chapter 7

THE PATIENT ENCOUNTER

Key Chapter Lessons

> Calculate your physician and staff time per minute

> Realize the dangers of batching work – and how to avoid it

> Understand how a virtual exam room can eliminate physicians' batching

> Learn the most effective steps to prepare for an encounter

> Recognize the value and components of pre-visit planning

> Understand the pitfalls of "service recovery" time

> Adopt a flow sheet to streamline the clinical area

> Identify the characteristics of efficient physicians

> Facilitate your patients' interaction with your practice

> Enhance patient-physician communications

> Recognize the importance of the tone set by the physician

Advanced Concepts

> Operations gap analysis

> The patient as co-producer

The actual encounter

The previous chapter explained how to process patients out of the "waiting" room quickly, or at least make their wait as pleasant as possible.

The next step in patient flow – the actual encounter between the patient and the physician – is the most important step in the entire process. The physician needs every tool possible to make this interaction friendly yet efficient, as well as to enable her to deliver the highest quality of care.

Make the most of the physician's time during the patient visit

Have you ever been focused on completing a complex task but then forced to put everything aside to search for a tiny piece of important information you need to finish? And did you also have 10 other tasks waiting at the same time? Now you know why physicians feel so frustrated when the patient flow process is inefficient and impedes their productivity. Sometimes, the interruption or logjam is missing information needed to refer a patient to the proper facility for a test, or a nurse who can't be immediately located to complete an exam.

Add all those extra minutes here and there that a physician spends each day tracking down some paperwork before, during or after a patient visit. Now, multiply those minutes by what the physician's time costs per minute. Beginning to see why patient flow problems can cost a medical practice big bucks?

How much does your physician's time cost?

It's pretty easy to find out what it costs your practice per minute of physician's time and identify when your physician is not providing care or engaged in related clinical activities.

In order to demonstrate, let's assume the following:

Physician compensation: $200,000

Physician weeks worked per year: 48

Physician hours worked per week: 55

55 hours (physician hours a week)* 60 minutes
= 3,300 minutes per week

3,300 minutes per week * 48 weeks (physician weeks a year)
= 158,400 minutes per year

$200,000 (annual physician compensation) / 158,400 minutes
= $1.26 per minute or $75.76 per hour

Now work through this formula using numbers from your own practice:

a = Annual physician compensation (_____)

b = Physician weeks worked per year (_____)

c = Physician hours worked per week (based on patient/physician interaction or communication; include operating room time for surgeons) (_____)

Step 1: c * 60 minutes = d (minutes per week)

Step 2: d * b = e (minutes per year)

Step 3: a / e = cost per minute

Note: Work through this formula for all the members of your staff who assist in the patient flow process

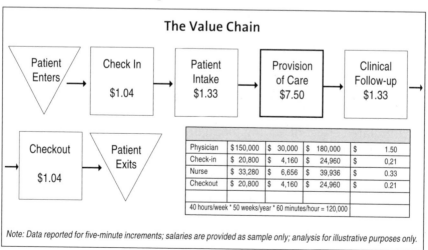

The Value Chain

Physician	$150,000	$ 30,000	$ 180,000	$	1.50
Check-in	$ 20,800	$ 4,160	$ 24,960	$	0,21
Nurse	$ 33,280	$ 6,656	$ 39,936	$	0.33
Checkout	$ 20,800	$ 4,160	$ 24,960	$	0.21

40 hours/week * 50 weeks/year * 60 minutes/hour = 120,000

Note: Data reported for five-minute increments; salaries are provided as sample only; analysis for illustrative purposes only.

The "per minute" cost has been calculated for each staff member assisting in the patient flow process. Note the difference between the cost of your staff and your physicians.

Stop all that batching

Although the cost of staffing each function before, after, and even during the patient encounter is lower than the physician's time, it's not a license for staff to be unproductive. Indeed, making each function work well is the key to streamlining patient flow. Unfortunately, a key ingredient to preventing productivity – batching work – is well entrenched at many practices.

Batching work – putting it off or organizing it to work on later – is sometimes appropriate but it has become an unhealthy addiction in some practices. It is much more efficient to process work on a real-time basis.

Take a hard look at how work gets done at your practice. Identify where work is batched and find a way to do it more quickly.

Set priorities. Some practices set specific hours for staff to work on certain tasks. For example, between 7:30 a.m. and 8:00 a.m., the medical assistant reviews the laboratory results from the prior evening. Abnormals are flagged and can be presented to the physician. At 8:00 a.m., he is ready to assist the physician in clinic. Then, from 1:00 p.m. to 1:30 p.m., while the physician is in with a patient for a procedure, the morning laboratory results are reviewed. This strict time allocation may not be appropriate for your practice but some staff may need assistance in setting priorities – and even when to get things done.

Review your systems and processes. Double-checking, intricate filing systems and other workflow tactics can make sense, but the accumulated effect of adding too many steps to the workflow can be disastrous. Review which steps in your work process are required and which ones just delay everyone from working on the task.

While super-organized processes boost efficiency, if taken too far, they can turn staff into full-time organizers who never get around to working. Take a step back and make sure the real work is getting done.

Make sure that you are not forcing staff to spend more time organizing work than they spend actually doing the work.

A virtual exam room

Staff aren't the only batchers. Physicians who stay late every night to return phone calls or complete documentation are probably batching too much work themselves. Guide them into the habit of stopping after every third or fourth appointment to spend a few minutes in a "virtual exam room" to complete the work that has built up.

It's quite tempting for physicians to batch their administrative work – reviewing messages, filling out forms, signing documents, making calls and dictating – until the end of the day. They want to focus entirely on seeing patients during office hours. You know who these physicians are in your practice because they are the ones who stay until 7:00 p.m. or later every night trying to dig out from the mountain of paperwork.

Practices are dealing with this problem by adding a virtual exam room. The exam room has nothing to do with adding floor space to your office. It is a concept designed to help physicians develop better work habits.

After every third or fourth patient, an appointment in the virtual exam room is designated just for the physician to deal with documentation, returning telephone calls or handling other quick tasks. The appointment may actually be scheduled in the system, or it may just be integrated into the flow. Either way, it means stopping to handle the work that has just come in during the last 30 minutes to an hour.

Physicians who hold all of those tasks until the end of the day will end up spending more time to get the tasks done, go home later and clog up the workflow for everyone.

Batching is destructive to efficient work and increases stress on physicians because it:

- Requires physicians to spend more time trying to "recall" the details of a patient visit while dictating;

- Leaves the physician with limited staff assistance during clinic because the staff is spend time fielding calls from anxious patients and referring physicians. The callers will continually call until they receive the information that is in limbo because the physician has batched his administrative tasks until the end of the day;

- Cause staff to spend more time organizing and managing telephone requests and callbacks; and

- Disrupts workflow by making staff begin each day dealing with the pile of work the physician left on their desks from the previous night.

Practices that use the virtual exam room concept find that they start and end their days on time. That is, physicians can actually start seeing patients at 8:00 a.m. as scheduled because their staff is ready to assist them, instead of trying to catch up work left over from yesterday.

CASE STUDIES

Practice uses the virtual exam room

Internal Medicine Associates realized that each of its physicians spent up to two hours a day on "paperwork." That is, their office hours were from 8:00 a.m. to 5:00 p.m., but the physicians were busy from 8:00 a.m. to 7:00 p.m. because they were dictating, responding to telephone calls, refilling prescriptions, completing paperwork, reviewing lab results and so on at the end of each day.

The physicians decided to stop batching work and try the virtual exam room. They added five minutes to each patient's visit. The extra time allowed the physicians to be more efficient by completing each patient's visit before the next patient arrived. When a patient left, the paperwork was complete, the prescriptions called in to the pharmacy and the clinical note dictated. Without decreasing the number of patients seen, the physicians found themselves out of the office by 5:30 p.m., instead of the inevitable 7:00 p.m. exit each evening.

Pre-visit planning

Preparing for the visit is important to keep workflow on track. Without pre-visit planning, chaos reins – and staff deal with it by trying to control it. This forces staff to batch work throughout the day. To avoid this non-value-added batching of work and foster real-time work processing, take the time to plan your day. You'll avoid the chaos — and reap the rewards of an efficient patient flow.

Pre-visit planning should start a day or two before the patient's scheduled appointment with these three steps.

Step One: Chart preview. A nurse or medical assistant should check the patient's medical chart before the visit. Regardless of whether the chart is a paper folder or an electronic medical record, it should be up-to-date with the patient's latest test results, hospital discharge summary, operative report, notes from a consulting specialist, and so on. If the results are not in the chart, get on the phone and obtain them. Have them faxed or e-mailed, or find them online.

If the physician requested a test or other referral that has not been completed, flag the chart for discussion with the physician on the day or two prior to the appointment. Evaluate whether the appointment should be rescheduled for a later date. If, for example, a patient was coming in to review the results of his liver biopsy, and the biopsy hasn't even been performed, then it's a waste of the physician's – and the patient's – time to keep the appointment.

Also flag important reading pre-visit material, such as abnormal results that may have just come and must be presented to the patient at his appointment.

A physician who appears unaware of test results, consults, and other medical care to which she directed the patient will give the patient a negative impression. Even if a nurse is called in to the exam room to retrieve the results and they are found during the encounter, the scene will inevitably leave the patient wondering just what other important information may be in limbo.

To make chart previewing easier, have the physicians state – or repeat a summary of – their orders at the end of their dictation. That way, the nurse can just look back to the last dictation to ensure that she is capturing everything needed for the visit that is being previewed.

In addition to looking for records of past care, anticipate the physician's needs for the upcoming encounter. If the patient is making a follow-up visit, make sure the file folder (if you are using a paper record) contains all forms needed for that type of follow-up. This would include order forms for ancillaries, educational materials, pre-operative instructions, and so on. Do the same electronically if using an electronic medical record. Go ahead and complete any appropriate standard information on the forms (patient's name, account number, date of service, etc.).

Although staff may complain that this preview process is unnecessary and takes too much time, the work is being done anyway. That is, they're finding the test results, hospital discharge summary, forms, etc., but it's done in the middle of a busy clinic. More importantly, if staff waits until the physician discovers a missing result, it will slow down the physician's productivity significantly. Without a preview process, the physician cannot be efficient.

Step Two: Room stock. Pre-visit planning should also include stocking the exam room with all supplies that will be needed. Stock at the start of each day and check in between patient visits. The exam rooms should be stocked for the types of patient visits that the physicians in your practice typically handle. Previewing charts daily can determine if an exam room needs extra equipment or supplies.

The most efficient physicians never leave their exam rooms during the encounter. Why? Because they have the tools they need to get the job done!

Step Three: Huddle. Pre-clinic huddles that include the physician, nurse or medical assistant, and appointment scheduler should be held before each morning and afternoon clinic. This three- to five-minute informal chat is a time to quickly review the upcoming appointment schedule. Use the appointment schedule as the "agenda." The purpose of the huddle is to give everyone a rundown of what's going to happen that session or day and any important issues that may impact on the day's patient flow. Staff should note if there is anything out of the ordinary or any issues that must be resolved immediately. For example, if three new patients were accidentally booked for the same slot, determine which patients can be rescheduled. It's also a good time to alert the physician to things that might throw off the whole day, such as the mother who typically schedules an appointment for one child yet brings in her other children, too. By pulling all of the children's charts, the physician and staff are better prepared. Finally, this is an opportune time for the physician to note where patients could be squeezed in for acute problems, if necessary.

Make sure these briefings start on time, never run long and are mandatory. Otherwise, it's another meeting.

The pre-clinic huddle is like a football team getting ready for its next play. If every player is well-informed, the play will be executed effectively. Consider every clinic your "play;" if you're not coordinated, you'll never make a touchdown. Granted, even a huddle won't guarantee a touchdown (or an easy day), but you will be able to execute the play – instead of sitting back and waiting for the chaos to overwhelm you.

What's the real reason you're here?

Finding out the real reason for the patient's visit can help the physician better prepare for the appointment. A handy way to do this is to have schedulers ask patients to describe their major symptoms when they call for appointments. The schedulers also can ask, "Since the doctor wants to make sure he has enough time with you; can you tell us why you're coming in?"

Stagger lunch breaks so there is always a live operator to answer the telephone. Lunch operators may be the only time a patient can call. Some people do not have a private place to call from work and do not want to discuss medical problems in front of co-workers.

Previewing charts, stocking exam rooms and huddling twice a day will help your practice function efficiently. Plan for the visit: control the day before it controls you.

Service recovery

Unconvinced about the need to reduce your waiting time to improve patient service? Consider the amount of visit time that is consumed when a physician walks into the exam room and must deal with a patient who is frustrated by an hour-long wait. One multispecialty practice measured its "service recovery" time to be three minutes per visit. Discuss this in your own practice; it may compel you to work on reducing waiting times.

When the physician waits

As we learned from the prior value-chain exercise, the biggest hit on a medical practice's financial status comes from wasting the physician's time. Every additional minute that a physician spends trying to locate a nurse to wrap up a patient visit, locate a referral form and find a chart is not just time wasted: it's money down the drain.

Of course, no one wants to work in or be a patient of a medical practice where physicians step out of their exam rooms and holler for their nurse to get there "on the double!" So, pressuring the physician to speed things up is not really the way to go either. Instead, look for ways that physicians and all of their support clinical and non-clinical staff can work smoothly without creating conflicts or wasting the physicians' time.

One way to improve the flow process of the patient-physician encounter is to develop a "flow sheet." A flow sheet can capture most of the verbal communication that physicians rely on and, often, have to wait for.

Designed to capture communication regarding orders between the clinical team, the flow sheet should be designed to meet the needs of your practice. Consider the communications that take place in the hallway: "draw some blood on this patient," "let's send him down for a chest x-ray," etc.

Put these communications on a form that can stick to the record (sticky notes), and are printed in a bright color to be easily distinguishable. You can even print the flow sheets on two-ply paper, allowing the form to become a lab request form or to be given to patients with instructions. I'm not advocating the elimination of all verbal communication, only to streamline flow.

Sample Flow Sheet

Flow Sheet

Date: _____ RTX: _____

PATIENT NAME: _____

DX: _____

MEDS:

_____

LABS

_____

EKG	❑	SIGMO	❑
GUAIAC	❑	PSA	❑
MAMM	❑	XRAY	❑
PAP	❑	BLOOD	❑
BX	❑	CULT	❑
CALL PT	❑	COPY REC	❑

Rooming standards

In addition to communicating about the flow, it's important to have designated rooming or intake standards for your most common diagnoses. The rooming or intake process is the process whereby the nurse or medical assistant escorts a patient back to the exam room. In addition to the escort, this is the opportunity for the nurse or medical assistant to gather information about the patient to help the physician be more efficient during the encounter. If the vitals and history are recorded, for example, the time the physician needs to document the encounter can be lessened — and she can jump right into the assessment and plan.

To determine your most common diagnoses, begin by pulling a report from your practice management system with the top 10 diagnosis codes billed during the last year (based on volume). Gather the clinical team and discuss the preparations necessary for each diagnosis to streamline the clinical process. For example, weight might not be gathered for all patients, but it must be measured for prenatal patients in an obstetrics practice. Decide what needs to be done and where to record it.

When you are evaluating your rooming process, make sure that you are respecting your patients' privacy. Don't, for example, have three scales lined up in a sub-waiting area for everyone to watch patient weigh-in. Although you may have to balance equipment costs or staff time, it's important to maintain your patients' privacy – and their dignity.

Revisit your rooming criteria every year. Even if your staff "knows" what to do, it doesn't hurt to discuss it periodically to accommodate different criteria for new services or physicians, as well as to reinforce its importance to staff.

Practice solves ancillary results tracking frustration

One neurosurgery practice developed a two-ply 3x5 card to order a MRI. The physician completes the card, and the medical assistant processes the request. Prior to submitting the request to radiology, a copy of the request is removed and filed in a box in date order. As the findings are reported, the copy of the request is removed from the box. Every week, one MA is assigned to review the requests that have not been read. This same system can be integrated with the "flow sheet."

For more ideas regarding monitoring test results, see Chapter 8, "Checkout."

The efficient physician's primer

Staff do not have the only role in making the patient encounter efficient. Following are steps that today's most efficient physicians complete each day to see more patients without staying later at work or taking administrative work home:

Review the next day's schedule by 3:30 p.m. each day. Look for mistakes. Note any changes and give them to the front office by 4:00 p.m. so staff can immediately contact affected patients to reschedule. If the scheduling process works well (see Chapter 4, "Scheduling," for tips on enhancing your scheduling), these changes should be minimal.

Huddle with your core staff before each clinic session *everyday*. Never skip this meeting. Go over any changes or mistakes in the schedule, chronic no-shows on the schedule, messages that are expected and how they should be handled. Involve the scheduler in the huddle or give any changes to the front office staff immediately.

Stay on time. Empower support staff to help. Many physicians set their pager on vibrate-only mode and ask support staff to page them when they are with a patient for more than a specified period of time, such as 30 minutes. Or, staff are instructed to interrupt with the statement: "Dr. Jones is on the phone for you." The physician can ignore the signal that it's time to move on or use it as a polite excuse to wrap up.

Pull work into the day. Use the virtual exam room, which is previously discussed in the Advanced Concepts section in this chapter, to avoid it piling up for later.

Start on time. If you don't start the day on time, don't expect to run on time. Many physicians start late because of the scheduling system. The appointment schedule is formulated to create a problem. For example, the first appointment is at 8:00 a.m. The patient has to pass through check-in, registration and the rooming process before being read for the physician. Even in the most efficient practices, this occurs often 15 or even 30 minutes after the patient has arrived. Set your schedule accordingly – if you want your physician to start at 8:00 a.m., have the first appointment scheduled at 7:30 or 7:45 a.m.

Standardize exam rooms. Have equipment, forms, computer terminal, and so forth in the same place so that you don' t have to think twice when reaching for something. Moreover, with standard exam rooms, physicians can use any exam room in the practice, if necessary.

Match young physicians with a "mentor." Help them adjust to your practice and establish expectations. Residency programs are notorious for failing to teach their trainees anything about efficiency. It's important to train physicians about efficiency before bad work habits set in.

Keep your team on the same page. For example, maintain a written log of scheduled patients at the nurses' station; as a patient is roomed, mark the exam room number next to the patient's name, and check off the patient as the visit is completed or the appointment is cancelled.

Stay focused. Limit interruptions during clinic, such as prolonged conversations with pharmaceutical sales representatives or telephone calls to your financial advisor. Schedule time for these before or after clinic.

Document during the visit. Dictate during the visit or at least after every third visit if using the virtual exam room concept. It's more efficient than batching dictation until the end of the day or the end of the week. (For more information on efficient decumentation, see Chapter 8, "Checkout.")

Set priorities. Days are long in a medical practice and it's easy to get buried in the details. That's why some physicians carry a laminated picture of their family in a shirt pocket. Each time there is an extra chore, they can pull out the picture and ask: "Can I delegate this task to support staff so that I can continue with the day and get home sooner?"

Efficient physicians are centered people. They don't get trapped in their practices. They know that their patients may love them but studies show that many patients will switch to other physicians over as little as a $10 dispute. They know that caring for patients doesn't mean abandoning one's personal or family life. Be good to yourself and you can be good to your patients.

Inefficiency: A vicious spiral

A little inefficiency can quickly lead to big problems. If you're struggling with inefficiency, see if this scenario sounds familiar:

Dr. Jones struggles to keep up with his patient volume, and work begins to pile up. Messages come in, prescription refills are requested, and forms stack up. In between rooming patients, his nurse, Judy, spends time organizing the growing stack.

By 5:30 p.m., clinic is winding down. Dr. Jones tells Judy to head home; she already has worked a half hour of overtime. Judy shows him the messages and paperwork that needs attention and leaves.

Alone, Dr. Jones begins the paperwork by returning calls to patients – though the nurse could have returned the call had Dr. Jones instructed her to earlier in the day. He leaves notes to Judy about the messages that can wait for morning, the refills, and the forms by sticking eight notes to Judy's chair and stacking a pile of charts on the counter for her to handle the following morning.

Office hours start again at 8:00 a.m., and Judy makes it to the office five minutes early. She puts her personal items on her desktop, and looks at the notes stuck to her chair and the charts spilling over her desk.

Here's where the inefficiency becomes a vicious spiral: Would any nurse in her right mind ignore the charts, and walk to the reception area to escort the first patient in to an exam room? Of course not. Faced with the pile of charts, Judy will easily spend at least the first 30 minutes of the day handling a portion of them. Of course, in the meantime, today's messages, forms, refills and other paperwork start to filter in. She is handling yesterday's *and* today's work. Her anxiety level increases, and her morale decreases. It's not hard to conclude that Judy's productivity, in turn, declines.

Thus, it's no surprise that the first patient isn't ready for Dr. Jones until 8:45 a.m. The day is running late already.

A little inefficiency soon leads to a problem with staff productivity and turnover, and negatively impacts patient satisfaction as well. It also means, as well, that the physician is rarely home before his spouse and children are asleep.

If you're in the vicious cycle of inefficiency, it's important to recognize it won't get better until you take concrete steps to stop the cycle. Implement efficiency strategies before you find yourself and others around you burned out.

Quality, not quantity is the key to a successful visit

I'm sure that there is at least one physician in your community with a terrific reputation among patients – yet it is rumored that the same physician can see 40 or more patients a day and still finish on time. These physicians have a special gift for getting the work done faster — while making the patient perceive the visit was longer. That is, a patient leaves with the impression that the physician spent an hour with him while the encounter was actually only six minutes. These special physicians may have personality traits that help them, but don't despair. There are still some characteristics that you can learn from these naturally efficient physicians — and adopt for yourself.

Here are techniques that the most efficient (and popular) physicians use to keep patients happy and practice revenue flowing:

Make eye contact. Eye contact indicates interest and creates a connection between the physician and the patient.

Sit with the patient. Physicians who stand during a discussion with a patient may convey that they are in a hurry. Sitting down indicates an interest in what the patient has to say.

Reach out to the patient. It doesn't have to be a physical touch; just an introduction and a smile will work. A handshake or a gentle touch when, and if, appropriate during the encounter can go a long way.

Make chitchat. A few friendly words regarding the patient's family or work gets the visit off to a friendly start and doesn't have to eat up precious time. As noted previously, some physicians keep personal notes in the patient's chart as a reminder.

Make sure the patient is comfortable. A patient who has been sitting in a chilly exam room for 30 minutes – naked, save a piece of paper wrapped around their hips – is not going to be in the best of moods when you enter. Make sure your patient is comfortable, and you won't have to spend the first few minutes of the encounter "warming" the patient up. Try upgrading to linen gowns – available in regular and extra-large sizes – to help you and your patients.

Listen first. Studies show that patients start off by discussing their least important complaints and build to the more intimate or distressing symptoms. Physicians who let the patient finish talking, while making notes or jotting down questions, get through interviews faster and make patients feel as if they were heard.

The impact of poor communication skills

Research conducted by Peggy Choong, PhD, of Lewiston, NY-based Niagara University revealed that a physician's poor communication skills have more than 3.5 times the negative impact on patient satisfaction than any positive performance ratings of the same skills.

Do some work in front of your patients. Physicians can begin reviewing the patient's chart at the nurses' station or in the hallway but complete the review of the chart and any tests or lab results in the exam room with the patient. It's a good opportunity to educate the patient about what you're assessing, explain what the tests were for and what the results mean. Often, patients don't see this extra time that you spend managing their care. Do it in front of them and they'll realize their time with you is really 15 minutes – not five.

Be happy. If you're unhappy, everyone around you – including your patients – will feel this. Happy physicians are not just more pleasant, they are more productive because their staff and patients respond to their optimism.

Although some physicians are naturally gifted with good – and efficient – bedside manners, it is possible for these characteristics to be learned.

A personal touch

Patients are delighted when their physician remembers personal information about them. This personal touch not only represents great service – it can foster efficiency. Physicians will appear distant and, perhaps, unsympathetic when they can't recall important pieces of information that a patient may have mentioned either to the physician on a previous visit or to some other member of the staff. If they do remember, patients feel a connection to their physician earlier in the encounter. Establishing an instant rapport with the patient delights them — and lets the physician walk out of the exam room having gathered and discussed more information in a shorter period of time.

A little advance work by the staff can help bring busy physicians up-to-date on their patients and immediate families. Delineate a place in your patients' charts to note personal topics, like profession, spouse's name, and even hobbies. Or, record a line in the dictation of the encounter. So, if the patient brings you a small gift, like a book, you can tell him how much you have enjoyed the book when they returns for the next appointment.

Some practices even have staff review the local newspaper on a daily basis, clip out any articles that mention or relate to their patients, and file or scan them into the appropriate patients' charts.

As with medical information, it's important to respect the patient's privacy, so keep all non-public information confidential.

Reach out to patients now, not later

The telephone is a wonderful time-saver, but it is not always the ideal way to communicate important information to patients. Instead of spending time trying to track down patients after their appointment by telephone and risking the compromises in confidentiality that come with electronic communication, why not try to communicate as much information to patients during the visit? It will save you time in the long run.

Here is a checklist of information that every patient should be able to receive during her visit:

❑ When and how they will receive their test results?

❑ When and for what purpose is the next visit to be scheduled?

❑ What is the diagnosis (presented such that patients can understand)?

❑ What is the treatment plan?

❑ How and where can the patient receive additional educational information related to the complaint/diagnosis(es)?

❑ If applicable, written orders for employer (e.g., return to work), prescriptions, etc.

Improve patients' retention of information

Studies have shown that patients only retain part of the information that is communicated during the encounter. Although it may be routine for your practice, most patients are surprised to hear that a procedure or surgery is in order. Shocked by the news, they often do not hear anything else you tell them.

When patients don't remember what the physician explained, they are more likely to call the practice when they return home. This, of course, requires that you dedicate staff time in answering these telephone calls. If you can communicate better with patients during the face-to-face encounter, you can avoid some, if not all, of these calls.

Give the patient written material about their condition or procedure, or write out the patient's treatment plan on paper or even a flipchart. Direct them to specific Web sites for more information or support groups. Customize a Web site for each patient.

When there is something more complicated at hand, say a surgery, some physicians provide educational videotapes or software about the surgery, as well as pre- and post-operative information for patients.

Others use simpler technology, including paper and pencil, which can work just as well.

If patients do not speak English, or if it is a second language for them, it is still the physician's duty to make sure the patient understands what the physician says. Use of qualified interpreters or translated patient education materials may be necessary.

The flipchart tells the story

An oncologist in the southeast uses a flipchart to outline the treatment plan for patients. As he talks to a patient, the oncologist uses a colored marker to draw a quick and simple timeline of the treatment process on a flipchart. What patients really seem to value is that they can take the oncologist's chart home with them to keep. Many refer to it often.

Try video

Why not videotape the doctor? Patients scheduled for surgery or diagnostic procedures have a million questions – including some that they won't think of asking until they've already left the practice site. Since the physicians at your practice have most of the answers – and have heard most of the questions already – why not help your patients by videotaping the physician explaining the surgery itself and the follow-up procedure? It doesn't have to be a million-dollar video production. It can be a terrific time-saver, and patients will love you for it. To reduce worries about potential litigation, make sure you review this project and the script with your attorney. Or, consider an educational tape published by your specialty society or another legitimate source.

Handling the "oh, by the ways"

Despite your best efforts to improve your work style, you may find your newfound efficiency backsliding at the sound of four little words – "oh, by the way...". You may even have your hand on the door ready to leave, and this short but powerful statement sends a shudder down your spine as you turn around to hear the rest of the story. It may be a patient with a minor question or comment but it's often a major issue.

Urologists, for example, find this to be commonplace. Male patients often leave questions about impotence until the end of the visit. They're embarrassed about it, but can't face their wives in the waiting room who will surely ask, "Did you talk to the doctor about *the* issue?" as soon as they see them.

The "oh, by the ways" can lead into an extended office visit that will put an already late physician further behind schedule. If you often hear the four little words, don't lose hope. There are strategies to help you:

Develop a better scheduling script. Instruct schedulers to get more information from patients when they set up appointments. For example, schedulers can say, "The doctor wants to have enough time to meet your health care needs; is there anything else that you want to discuss with her?" It won't work every time but setting expectations upfront never hurts.

Postpone the concern. If the patient's last-minute concern is complex, there is nothing wrong with asking him to schedule another appointment. For example, the physician can say, "This is an important discussion and I want to make sure we give enough time to it. Since we made time today to address only your XYZ concern, I'd like to schedule another visit with you so we can have enough time to address this." Have patient education material ready for frequently asked questions so patients don't go home empty-handed.

Preempt. Address common questions before patients bring them up. For example, expect that a post-menopausal woman will ask questions about hormone replacement therapy. Have written material on hand and direct the patient to Web sites that meet the physicians' approval. The physician can offer a brief summary of advice and ask a nurse or medical assistant to discuss the issue further with the patient to see if another appointment is needed.

Recognize that there are communication differences in male and female patients. Male patients often leave the most important issues until the end. To avoid this, draw the information out early with open-ended questions and proactively inquire about sensitive issues that are relevant to the patient's encounter.

Seize the opportunity. Sometimes, dealing with the "oh by the way" comment today heads off more work tomorrow. For example, it may be possible to add a routine exam to an already scheduled follow-up visit which will open the physician's schedule to accommodate another patient. This strategy won't make sense if the extra work adds no additional reimbursement, creates inconvenience for the patient or puts the physician behind schedule.

Learn to code. Physicians who understand evaluation and management coding and the proper use of modifiers to indicate extra work can accommodate last-minute questions during patient encounters and get paid what they deserve. If you can't control the "oh, by the ways," at least get paid for them.

Medical schools getting on the communications bandwagon...finally

Some medical schools are paying more attention to training new physicians in the art of communications. As a volunteer for a medical school, I was assigned to role-play a patient who was receiving post-biopsy results that unfortunately determined a malignant carcinoma. In this exercise, the physician (played by a medical student taking the course) bravely told the author just what the lab results stated: "malignant carcinoma of the spleen." Considering the fourth-grade reading level of the majority of U.S. citizens, many patients would have walked away with this dreadful news without really knowing how serious the problem was, other than it involved the spleen (whatever that was).

This type of miscommunication is even more serious due to the fact is that many patients don't ask sufficient follow-up questions because they fear appearing ignorant. When answering patient's questions, physicians should be coached to respond in the patients' non-technical language. Not only do miscommunications of this sort reduce the quality of care and seem to raise physicians' malpractice liability risks, they tend to increase the amount of work for the practice. Rest assured that when a patient doesn't understand what the physician said, it won't be long until the patient calls the office for better understanding of the situation.

The physician sets the tone

I was recently pulled aside by a productive family practitioner with more than 30 years of experience. He told me that he had *the* answer to physician efficiency.

"If I started complaining about appointments scheduled at 4:45 p.m., the employees would hear me. Even if I didn't ask for a different schedule, staff would stop filling the 4:45 p.m. slot. We'd all be home in time for dinner, but we'd lose money. Whether we acknowledge it or not, our staff is always listening," he said.

His lesson was simple, but incredibly powerful: the physician sets the tone for the practice.

It isn't just what you say at staff meetings, it's what physicians "say" to everyone in the office – staff, patients and other physicians – through their day-to-day actions. Whether or not the practice is physician-owned, the physician shapes the atmosphere and influences the long-term success of the practice.

Physicians who want to make their practices better places to work start with themselves.

Physicians put in long hours and work hard, and expect those around them to do the same. But if the physician comes back from lunch an hour late every day leaving an office full of frustrated patients, it won't take long for staff to replicate the pattern.

Physicians set the tone; a hard worker will usually end up with hard workers around them.

Efficient physicians look for solutions, not scapegoats. They seek out ways to improve performance. These physicians focus on the big picture. They do whatever it takes to create a culture of problem solving. They refuse to engage in the behind-the-scene gripe sessions and clique forming that are all too common in health care settings. When someone starts complaining about someone else, they simply change the topic. In time, that behavior earns the respect of peers and staff. Better yet, people spend more time thinking about patients and going home happy.

Although we often find excuses to blame the system (whatever that is), there is no one stopping you from creating an efficient patient encounter in your practice. Embrace change and you will find your patients, staff and even physicians more productive – and happier too!

ADVANCED CONCEPT

Operations gap analysis

Although you may be measuring patient satisfaction with the latest and greatest survey instrument, even the best patient satisfaction surveys have their limitations. How about doing an "operations gap analysis?" The results will prove much more valuable to the practice and its future direction.

An "operations gap analysis" is a complex term for a simple concept – survey your patients, employees and physicians with the same questions. Measure the patient results against the results you receive from your physicians and employees. The "gap" between the results of the groups is where you should focus future efforts to change.

Why focus on the gaps? Because the gaps between what your patients and what your staff or physicians think about an issue reveal important differences in perceptions. If your physicians and employees strongly feel that they're doing a great job on a certain process, then they will have no impetus to change the procedure or their behavior in doing it, no matter how low the patient satisfaction survey rates them. But showing them that gap in perception through hard data can change some minds.

By pinpointing the gaps in perceptions, the gap analysis survey will allow your practice to recognize what you think you are doing well and what you're not doing well, where you excel and where you need improvement. Don't ignore the areas where both sets of participants rate your practice's performance low.

The patient as co-producer

So far, we've focused on the physician as the main producer of revenue in the practice. Of course, that is true, but don't forget where that revenue really comes from: it comes from patients.

Many service industries realize that everything they do starts and stops with the customer. To gain maximum value from their interaction with their customer and give the customer a better experience — namely, more convenience at less cost — many service providers are integrating customers into their workforces. How? Consider these examples:

Industry customer turns provider through:

- Automated teller machines (ATM);

- On-line bill payment;

- Restaurants salad bars;

- Self-service cashiering at retail stores;

- Self-serve gasoline stations;

- Self-serve car washes;

- Self-serve parking lots; and

- Retail Internet "stores."

Well, okay, let's admit it, the customer is doing more of the work in one sense. But the return is (ideally) faster service, more convenience and lower cost. Putting the customer in charge can save the organization time and money, too.

Consider where this concept of "co-production" can fit into your practice's operations. How about:

- Placing pads of paper titled "Issues I wish to discuss with the doctor today" in the reception area. This may help save time at the beginning of the visit when the patients recall all of their symptoms.

- Providing patient education materials or videos to patients to view while waiting or after visits may answer many of the questions they might have asked and allow better use of the time they are with the physician.

- Allowing patients who have Internet access or e-mail to complete all of their paperwork before the day of the visit and submitting them in advance.

- Sending patients statements via e-mail and accepting payment online.

- Maintaining treatment plans or logs online for patients to record and even assess their own care with clinical algorithms.

Consider your patients as co-producers, and discover new and innovate ways that *they* can help you.

Chapter 8

CHECKOUT

Key Chapter Lessons

> Evaluate your checkout process

> Identify the various components of checkout

> Learn charge entry methodologies

> Recognize the most efficient process for follow-up scheduling

> Identify the pros and cons of processing referrals and appointments for ancillary services and specialists

> Track test results effectively

> Facilitate payment at checkout

> Learn to document more efficiently

> Learn about integrating "care teams" into your practice

Checkout checklist

- ❑ Do checkout staff get the information they need about the patients' follow-up visits so they don't have to depend on patients to tell them when they are to return?
- ❑ Are patients told what ancillaries are required?
- ❑ Are patients told where to go for their appointment(s)?
- ❑ Are patients told how and when they will be contacted regarding test results?
- ❑ Do patients feel that all of their questions have been answered?
- ❑ Are patients given the opportunity to provide input regarding their encounter (e.g., patient satisfaction survey)?
- ❑ Are fees collected in a courteous but firm manner?
- ❑ Can patients pay by cash, check, credit or debit card?
- ❑ How quickly are charges entered into the system?
- ❑ What steps are taken to ensure that charges are accurate?
- ❑ Is there some meaningful communication at patients' departures to conclude the visit?
- ❑ Do patients receive all of the educational materials that may be needed?
- ❑ Have patients had their prescription(s) refilled?

Save time and money at the end of the patient flow process

The checkout step of the patient flow process should complete the patient encounter, not extend it. Checkout also is a time for staff to anticipate and meet the patient's needs for additional information. The tasks included in the checkout process vary from practice to practice, but I'll review those functions common to most medical practices.

Smooth checkout saves time on the telephone

Want to reduce the volume of unnecessary telephone calls to the practice and the time staff spends handling those calls? Then, make sure patients get every piece of information they may need before they leave the practice after their visit is concluded. When a patient has to call back for more information after the visit, staff time is spent locating the file, researching the proper answer and, possibly, checking with a member of the clinical staff to make sure the right information is being provided. To reduce the volume of unnecessary callbacks, make sure that each departing patient gets the following information at checkout:

- Follow-up scheduling
- Outbound referrals and ancillaries
- Payments
- Educational materials
- Prescriptions

If there is information that is given out routinely, to include appointment reminders, prepping instructions for procedures, and directions to lab or imaging facilities, create pre-printed materials to use.

I'll first begin with the charge entry process, which typically occurs at checkout.

Charge entry

The most effective way to ensure that no encounter forms (also known as charge tickets or superbills) are misplaced is to make sure that staff at the checkout counter or area collect 100 percent of them at the conclusion of the patient's visit. But to make this happen, physicians must complete their patients' charge tickets at the end of each visit, not at the end of the day. Capturing all services accurately is of primary importance for proper billing and reimbursement. If charge tickets aren't complete when the patient is ready to go, they must be collected retrospectively and that's where costly mistakes and delays can occur.

Accuracy or timeliness?

For charge capture, accuracy is paramount. If you have to choose between the accuracy and timeliness of charge entry, choose accuracy.

Two ways to handle charge tickets at checkout

Charges can either be keyed in or batched at checkout:

Keying In: Charges are keyed into the practice management system as patients exit or as time permits during the day. If the charge tickets are accurate (that is, all charges have been recorded and are appropriate), keying in at checkout is the most efficient way to enter charges. As I have discussed in other chapters, real-time processing of work is the most efficient.

Batching: Charge tickets are gathered and stacked. Near the end of the session, the tickets are checked over and batch totals are run. The process typically includes summing up the charges and payments attached to the charge tickets (that is, the time-of-service payments) and recording the count on a standard batch cover sheet. Many groups attach the printout from a calculator to the cover sheet. As with keying in, accuracy is of primary importance.

Either way, a real-time charge editing system that interfaces (or is integrated) with your practice management system will allow you to create a more accurate claim. (Accuracy cannot be guaranteed because of the proprietary edits used by insurance companies that can change on an almost daily basis.) This system can give you real-time feedback regarding charges that were posted inaccurately by having imbedded logic regarding the appropriate use of coding and modifiers. With an editing system, you can fix the problem on a real-time basis, alleviating the re-work that occurs in the billing office (and often comes back to the physician to fix).

If automation is not an option for you due to the lack of products or money, then create your own charge editing process. Train the checkout staff in coding or have a member of the billing office who works insurance claims review the charges manually.

Follow-up scheduling

The encounter form should include a place for the physician to indicate the time a patient is requested to return for another visit (e.g., "two weeks" or "four months"), if one is necessary. The checkout staff can utilize this information to offer a date(s) and time(s) for the patient to return to the practice for the follow-up visit. Once the date and time are chosen, offer the patient some written confirmation of the appointment by printing a confirmation from the system or writing the appointment details on a pre-printed appointment reminder card.

Scheduling Follow-up Appointments

Frustrated by the volume of patients that slams your practice each week? Smooth demand by scheduling all follow-up visits on Tuesday through Friday (unless the patient requests a Monday). When a physician indicates a follow-up visit to be scheduled in four weeks, request that your checkout clerk looks for an appointment slot that does not fall on a Monday. This policy will allow you to keep Mondays primarily available to acute visits, which should make your Mondays much more manageable.

When scheduling patients for follow-up at the time of checkout, be sure to maintain scheduling templates at least three months out. A shorter timeframe will cause your checkout staff to request that the patient "just give us a call." By processing the work on a real-time basis, your practice can reduce telephone demand.

Delaying the appointment scheduling process will require your staff to spend more time accommodating the patient because the scheduler will have to ask the patient to repeat the physician's instructions for a follow-up visit, chief complaint, etc. The only word of caution is that scheduling too far out will create no-shows because patients are likely to forget an appointment they scheduled 12 months ago. There's no hard and fast rule, but it's generally not a good idea to schedule more than six months out.

See Chapter 4, "Scheduling," for more tips about appointment scheduling.

Outbound referrals and ancillaries

At the end of the encounter, the physician may decide to refer the patient to a specialist(s) and/or for an ancillary service(s). Depending on the patient's insurance, a referral may also need to be processed. Processing referrals usually consists of obtaining an authorization from the patient's insurance company that a test, consult or other service can be made. Ancillary services, such as physical therapy or MRI, almost always require a written request from the referring physician as well as an approval from the insurance company. Because outbound referrals are generally required for ancillary services, these processes are described together. No matter what paperwork is involved, this process can be conducted in any of four ways, or some combination of them:

1. **Checkout counter referral and scheduling**: Patients who are to be referred to a specialist or to receive ancillary services are given the necessary paperwork in the exam room (or the instructions are

noted on the charge ticket or an internal routing form). The patient is directed to the checkout counter where a staff member (typically, a non-clinical administrative staffer) process the paperwork and/or schedules the appointment(s). Some of these functions can be set aside or batched later in the interest of the patient's time. However, if there is time, it is best for staff to call the physician, ancillary facility or other provider to whom the patient is being referred and make the necessary appointments for the patients. For a courtesy referral (e.g., an OB/GYN suggests a dermatologist to a patient who complains about post-partum hair loss), the patient may be requested to schedule the appointment herself.

Pros: The checkout function is completed in a single process. The patient is moved away from the clinical area without any further distraction to the physician.

Cons: The physician originating the request may have to provide additional information before the appointment can be made. If so, the checkout staff will have to leave the workstation and find the physician to get the necessary clarification.

It is generally not cost effective to employ staff with clinical training at a checkout desk. However, handling these requests does require some proficiency in clinical terminology to make sure the proper appointments are made with the appropriate providers. That may require staff members who have no clinical training to ask many questions of other staff and slow down the process in order to complete this step accurately and efficiently. A way around this is to hire a medical assistant or nursing assistant for the position.

Key referral concepts

Outbound Referrals: The practice refers the patient out of the practice to a specialty physician (e.g., orthopedic surgeon) or other services provided outside the practice (e.g., physical therapy). Outbound referrals are generally made by primary care physicians, but many specialists refer out for ancillary services and/or for consults with other specialists. Outbound referrals are processed at the end of the visit. They can be done in more than one way (see outbound referrals and ancillaries). This allows the patient to promptly receive information regarding the referral to another provider or facility.

Inbound Referrals: The practice accepts the outbound referral (as just described) from other practices. Inbound referrals are generally received by specialty physicians, and should be processed during check-in or preferably on a pre-visit basis; that is, the referring physician or patient should communicate the inbound referral prior to or at the time of the patient's visit. The referral is necessary for the specialty provider to receive appropriate payment.

To summarize: Outbound referrals are processed at the end of the visit or at checkout; inbound referrals are processed at check-in or preferably on a pre-visit basis. Outbound referrals are made to specialists or ancillary providers, and become inbound referrals for those same providers.

Another disadvantage of handling referrals and appointments at the checkout counter is that these counters are typically located where the patient's and staff member's conversations can be overheard by others, especially if there is a line of patients waiting to check out. Few practices can afford to have several semi-private counters as many hospital emergency rooms do for admissions.

An additional disadvantage is that patients typically want to leave as quickly as possible after they complete their visit. This method can lead to considerable queues, particularly if there is only one staff member handling checkout.

2. Exam room referral and scheduling: Conduct the referral and scheduling process in the exam room. It is certainly private, but a telephone or computer connection must be available for the staff member to use in securing the referral and/or making an appointment.

Pros: Work is processed on a real-time basis. A medical assistant or nurse can begin the process immediately after the visit is concluded or, possibly, before the physician has left the exam room. This method also allows for maximum privacy and confidentiality.

Cons: Exam room referrals tie up exam rooms. If space is at a premium in your practice and this method causes your physician to be idle while waiting for an available exam room, then think twice about using this process – a physician's time is the most expensive thing to waste in your practice.

3. Nurses' station referral and scheduling: Have a medical assistant or nurse conduct the referral and/or scheduling process at the nurses' station. A suitable telephone or computer connection must be available.

Pros: The clinical expertise of the medial assistant or nurse will be helpful to ensure an efficient referral or appointment scheduling process. From the nurses' station, a nurse or the physician can usually be located quickly if there are questions.

Cons: Nurses' stations are not the places to create lines of patients waiting to be served. You do not want patients hanging out in the clinical area if at all possible because this creates a distraction for the physicians and other patients. It increases the opportunities for a patient to waylay a physician to ask more questions and, potentially, impact the physician's productivity. Ideally, all of the patient's questions should have been answered during the clinical encounter.

Preparing the patient for the test

Some hospitals and testing facilities give practices the necessary items to prepare patients for their tests. With the preparatory materials on hand, the practice can then send patients directly to the testing facility. For example, the practice will have on hand oral contrast necessary for certain CT scans. Patients are given instructions to drink the contrast and directed to the testing facility. By the time that the patient reaches the facility, he's ready for the test.

4. Automated referral and scheduling: Technology may allow your practice to process most – if not all – referrals and authorizations automatically. Some insurance companies offer a portal through which to request and monitor referrals, and there are vendors who contract with insurance companies and practices to manage the same process for a fee. If you have an EMR, you could even automate the request process directly from the physician's orders.

Technology may also allow your practice to automate the scheduling of ancillary services and appointments with specialists. Many integrated health systems give their member practices access to schedule appointments online, or accept requests electronically at the offices of their ancillary facilities and specialists.

Or, you can program your own EMR to automate the paperwork for you and even send an electronic request automatically when the physician chooses to refer a patient for a test or to a specialist.

Pros: Automating the referral and scheduling process can improve workflow and eliminate staff time.

Cons: The technology to process the referrals and schedule the appointments may not be cost-effective or even possible at your practice. Your practice is at the mercy of the hospitals, laboratories, imaging facilities and specialists' offices – until they can accept and process the request automatically, you may be tied to the fax or the phone.

The best approach for handling referrals and appointments may be a hybrid model in which follow-up appointments and referrals are processed at checkout while all ancillaries and specialists' appointments are scheduled in the clinical area, either at the nurses' station or in an exam room, depending on the space and technology available. By using the time the patient is dressing after the exam, you can reduce the lines that are created by patients waiting and serve your patients promptly.

No matter where you do it, processing referrals and appointments can be an operational headache; deploy automation and technology in every way possible to streamline this process.

No more scheduling

If you have concerns about whether you are required to schedule the appointment(s) with facilities and specialists to whom you have referred your patients – and whether you have to make sure that they actually keep their appointment there – check with your malpractice carrier. Some practices have stopped scheduling appointments with testing facilities and specialists and just give instructions to patients to make their own appointments, but there may be risk management issues for you to consider depending on the situation.

Help your patients

If you are referring the patient for a test that requires preparation, be sure to give the patient instructions about preparing for the test. Give the patient a map to the facility if it's not at your practice's offices.

Test results

Whether you refer a patient to an external facility for a test or send the patient to your own ancillary services, you should have a mechanism in place to track the ordering and reporting of results for each test ordered.

There are many ways to monitor the testing and reporting process, but it's important to choose one method and follow it religiously. Even one lost test result can have serious implications for your patients' safety.

Some popular monitoring methods are:

Record the order. Although this may seem like a "no-brainer," practices sometimes schedule tests but fail to document the order. Or, the physician verbally tells the nurse or the patient to get the test but fails to document it in the patient's record. Develop a separate order form or create a template in your practice management system – or electronic medical record if you use one – to document all tests ordered.

Ask physicians to dictate information about any tests ordered into their documentation of the hospital or office visit. This note in the record will serve as a "tickler" that staff will see when they preview charts before the patient's next appointment. Thus, they know to look for the results. It should be noted that if a patient never has a return appointment, missing results may go undetected, so don't rely on this method to be fail-safe.

Keep a copy of each test order form in a date-ordered tickler file. Review this file daily to ensure that results are back when expected and that physicians are alerted.

Schedule a follow-up appointment to review test results one to two weeks after the patient's initial appointment. This is especially useful for biopsies, MRIs, CTs and other major tests where results should be delivered in person, not by mail or over the telephone. Staff are "tickled" or reminded that test results have arrived or will soon arrive during the chart preview process before the upcoming appointment. If the patient doesn't show up for the follow-up appointment, you'll be able to see that the patient still needs to be notified of the test results.

Hold patient charts in a special chart rack until the test results are in. Order the charts by the date the results are expected back. Review the rack daily for charts that remain there beyond the time that you expected the results to be returned.

Interface the reports from your in-house ancillaries and external providers with your EMR. Populate the relevant fields in the patients' chart with the results, and flag those charts for review.

Use your practice management system's "recall" function to prompt you for patients' test results. During checkout, for example, in addition to recalling a patient for her mammogram in the recommended number of months, input a recall to yourself that this year's mammogram is scheduled for next week and that you need to be "tickled" in two weeks for the test results.

Maintain a manual log of tests ordered. Keep the log at the nursing station, checkout counter or referral desk. The log should include a column titled "results back?". Highlight the appropriate entries as test results are received. Scanning the log daily for past entries that are not highlighted can alert you that a patient's test results have been delayed or lost.

Use a low-tech "to do" list in your PDA or desktop PC. In this slightly higher tech version of the manual log, you record test orders and patients' names in a to-do list in a spreadsheet or word processing program. Mark patients' names off as results are received. Check daily for names that remain on the list after results were expected. A simple calendar program, internal e-mail, or your scheduling module can serve the same purpose.

Utilize an automated lab results retrieval program. Integrate the software with your ancillary services or ordering process. Monitor un-retrieved results to alert you to a problem.

If you don't feel confident that your test tracking system works all the time, then tell your patients to call your practice if they haven't heard from you in a pre-determined time frame (e.g., two weeks). As mentioned in the chapter on telephones, this will increase your volume of incoming calls and increase the interruptions to staff as they track down results that may have not yet arrived or been reviewed by a physician. Keep in mind also that the "call us back in two weeks" solution often leaves the patient wondering whether your practice has the necessary systems to manage their care.

Awaiting test results can be a frightening experience for patients. To allay their fears – and reduce the amount of unproductive communication that takes place before tests results are confirmed – give patients written materials about their tests. Make sure the materials describe – in simple terms – what the test is for, why it is important for the physician to have the test and when to expect test results.

No matter what system you use, make sure that results are reviewed in a timely manner. Always communicate abnormal results immediately. And make sure that your tracking system – whether electronic or handwritten – is kept secure and can be accessed only by those in your practice who need to know the information.

No monitoring system is fail-safe. That's why you must hire employees who understand why medical tests are important. Staff your practice with employees who truly care about patients and you will already be well on your way to efficiently managing whatever process your practice puts in place.

Collection of payments

Checkout is the appropriate time to collect any monies owed to the practice if you have not collected payments prior to the time of service (at the front office). Be sure to request and collect these copayments, in addition to any co-insurance.

This is also a good time to ask for payment (in full or partial) on any outstanding account balances the patient may have from previous visits. Of course, this must be done in a polite, but appropriate manner. Staff may need a little training to hit the right balance of firmness and courtesy.

Don't wait until the checkout unless you have to; asking for payment can certainly be done at check-in.

Make sure your practice has the ability to accept credit cards, debit cards and personal checks, in addition to cash. If there are extenuating circumstances, such as patients who routinely write bad checks, then limit your options accordingly or take measures to prevent problems.

Don't rely on posted signs that say you "expect payment." Instead, instruct your staff to ask for payment politely but firmly, such as: "Ms. Smith, how would you like to take care of your charges with us today?"

More sophisticated practices are setting up payment plans at checkout, and some are even calculating the patient portion of the monies owed to the practice for services rendered (instead of waiting until insurance has paid), particularly in surgical practices.

Self-addressed envelopes

If patients don't have their payment available for what they owe to the practice, give them a self-addressed envelope to help make payment more convenient for them and more prompt for you.

Educational materials

If the physician or nurse has not done so already, provide education materials to patients at checkout according to their diagnosis. Unless the physician or nurse marks the appropriate materials (you can use a source number so that everyone in the practice will know that a "1" means the hypertension brochure, for example), consider having multiple pamphlets out for patients to chose themselves. It is important to handle this step carefully, you would not want the checkout staff to hand a patient the materials for a problem the patient doesn't even have.

Prescriptions

Ask patients if they have any questions about their prescriptions (new or refilled). If the practice has an automated prescription writer that prints at checkout, make sure that this process is facilitated.

Document encounters in real time

The documentation of the encounters doesn't occur at the checkout station – but it does occur after the encounter is complete. While the patient is being checked out, the physician is often in the back of the office documenting his encounter with the patient. If this isn't occurring – or you're looking for ways for the process to be more efficient, there's help for you.

Most practices have at least one physician in the practice who finds his schedule so overwhelming that the only time he can dictate notes is late at night or on his day off. If you can find ways for him to document more efficiently, you'll help your practice improve cash flow, reduce risk, improve patient care and lower the chances of physician burnout.

Yes, all physicians do get behind on documentation at times. But delaying dictation raises the likelihood that the physician might forget to document a provided service or procedure or note an important clinical question. The consequences can include increased chances of inaccurate coding and improper reimbursement – and the more serious malpractice consequence of failing to document an important finding or aspect of the treatment that compromises the future care of the patient.

Try these tips to help physicians who can't find time to document daily:

Develop documentation time savers. Ask the physician to write down the typical questions she asks of patients suffering from the five most common complaints she treats. Create a checklist of those questions with room for notes below each question. Based on the patient's chief complaint, put the appropriate template into the patient's chart when it's pulled for the next day's appointment. The checked-off items and notes on the template will help the physician save time later when dictating. Electronic medical records can automate this process – and make it more efficient – by electronically pulling templates and checklists based on the patient's risk factors and complaints.

Ask the physician to dictate notes more often. The most efficient time to dictate a note is after each patient or after every two or three patient visits at a maximum. With this information still fresh in mind, the physician spends much less time trying to remember or look up details about the patient's visit. Physicians who delay dictation until the evening or weekend will spend about 60 seconds to recall the relevant details and assemble the notes of each patient. For a daily workload of 25 to 30 patients, that can add 30 minutes to each day's dictation duties.

Dictate during the encounter. It is possible for physicians to document encounters in real time and do so in a patient-friendly way. The physician can explain that he is documenting the visit and would like the patient to hear what will be put into the record. The physician must not turn his back to the patient or mumble into the recorder. Few patients understand all of the medical terminology, but most will appreciate hearing the details of their visit and the plans for treatment. Dictating in front of the patient further reinforces the physician's assessment and plan, which can improve patient education and compliance.

Physicians who dictate in real time or after each patient visit are ready to focus on the next patient or task. And they have one less reason to feel overworked by long evening or weekend hours.

De-centralize checkout and use care teams

The checkout function varies according to specialty, but more practices are moving some, if not all, of the function physically closer to the clinical area and away from the check-in/reception area. This helps to more rapidly conclude the patient's visit without making the person wait in line at the front desk again.

"Care teams" can help handle the checkout process. These teams can be composed of a physician (or several), a clinical assistant (or several) and a member(s) of the clerical staff. The team's clinical members provide the care and, with the assistance of a trained member of the administrative staff (who can be a medical assistant, thereby allowing rotation of positions), explain follow-up activities to patients.

A more innovative approach translates this concept to a team who manages the patient encounter for its population of patients. For example, a greeter meets the patient upon arrival to the practice, verifying the information already collected by the registration staff on a pre-visit basis. The greeter prints the patient's charge ticket to the care team's pod. There, a patient flow coordinator picks up the charge ticket and the medical record (which was already pulled), walks to the reception area and escorts the patient back to the pod. The coordinator rooms the patient, and moves to prepare for the next encounter. A medical assistant works with the patient to take vitals and make preparations for the physician's visit according to the patient's chief complaint.

The physician enters, provides an assessment and diagnosis, then requests assistance from the medical assistant. After completing the visit, the medical assistant asks that the patient see the care team checkout clerk, who assists with making a follow-up appointment and any necessary paperwork. Another support staff answers phones for the care team, accepting appointment calls. The advantage? Staff members work side-by-side, eliminating the barrier between the "front" and the "back." Time dedicated to messaging reduces (because it can be managed on a real-time basis), and patients love the contact with a "team" rather than a faceless organization.

For more information about a similar concept called "pods," see Chapter 7: "The Patient Encounter."

Of primary importance in the care team approach is having a facility that supports the "team" structure. A facility with a tiny nurses' station and too few exam rooms will not allow for a decentralized checkout.

Don't try to decentralize if it compromises your practice's ability to collect payments at checkout or requires a multimillion-dollar investment for facility redesign. Before knocking down any walls, or giving up on the idea, try adding an administrative staff member to the nurses' station or at a small desk in a corner of the clinical area. You may discover that a de-centralized checkout is best for you and your patients.

A smooth and efficient checkout function allows your practice to complete the patient encounter on a positive note. Use this opportunity to leave an indelible positive impression of your practice on every patient.

Chapter 9

TECHNOLOGY

Key Chapter Lessons

> Recognize the key components of practice management systems

> Harnessing the Internet to work for you and your patients

> Integrate document management

> Learn about personal digits assistants (PDAs) and e-prescribing

> Recognize the benefit of an electronic medical record

> Understand how to prepare your practice for new technology

> Learn to evaluate technology purchases and to assess vendors

> Learn more than 30 ways to automate processes in your practice.

Technology offers bold innovation, but be careful to avoid obstacles

Buying the right information technology and using it correctly will make medical practice operations more efficient and effective. This chapter presents an overview of many technologies that can be used in medical operations, how to chose these technologies wisely and how to implement them successfully. It is not a primer on the hardware and software required to make your practice function; instead, this chapter will supplement your current knowledge and highlight the technology applications that can positively affect your practice operations.

The practice management system

Although there are still a few practices out there holding on for dear life to their pegboards and appointment books, most now have practice management systems that offer automated solutions for billing and accounts receivable, scheduling and registration. "Practice management system" is a catchall term. There are hundreds of practice management system vendors and many nuances to these systems. At the very least, make sure that your practice management system – or the next one you buy – can:

- Manage all of your billing and accounts receivable, scheduling, and registration functions;

- Share a master patient file with all its various modules to avoid re-keying;

- Transmit insurance claims and produce billing statements;

- Produce management reports;

- Allow upgrades to improve functionality and meet new regulatory and payer requirements; and

- Integrate with other software products and services – including those produced by other manufacturers.

Speaking of vendors, the company that sells you your new practice management system should be capable of providing more than a good product that works well for the moment. Since so much of your day-to-day operations will depend on the practice management system, it is wise to seek out a vendor that:

- Offers timely, accurate, accessible and cost-effective customer service;

- Supplies at no cost any updates or technical improvements necessary to fix system shortcomings or fix glitches;

- Produces upgrades that are reasonably priced and provide sufficiently improved functionality;

- Offers you ways to contact and share experiences with other users through users' conferences, networking groups and electronic mailing lists; and

- Responds appropriately and promptly to assure that the product — and the functions you perform with it — comply with new regulatory requirements, such as the Health Insurance Portability and Accountability Act (HIPAA).

Think of your technology vendors as important stakeholders in your practice's success.

Once you have chosen your core practice management system, your vendor can help you define your hardware needs. Be sure to revisit this topic every year to make sure that your hardware keeps up with the demands of your software.

The majority of practice management systems now in use are based on client-server technology. That is, you buy the system in a "box" and the software that makes it run resides in your practice. A growing number of medical practices are opting for systems that are Web-based or are provided by an application service provider (ASP) that is accessed via the Internet. There are many advantages to this model – the vendor tends to the software – but if you do, make sure that your vendor complies with current HIPAA regulations. Using ASP technology is acceptable under HIPAA. However, reasonable safeguards must be in place to ensure that your patients' information, the network connections between your practice and the ASP or Web-based service, and your practice management system itself are secure.

The Internet

New research indicates that the majority of patients access the Internet for information about their health. There's no restriction, and very little guidance, to help your patients differentiate between the many Web sites that provide accurate health information and the many more that do not. To help your lead your patients the best information on the Web, and make the Internet work for you consider:

- **Developing a Web site for your practice.** At minimum, include your practice's name, providers' names and backgrounds, practice location(s), driving directions, nearby public transportation if it is available in your community and who in your practice to contact for more information. Consider also putting your practice's policies for financial obligations, prescription refills, telephone calls and appointment scheduling on your Web site;

- **Directing patients to Web sites approved by your physicians.** Develop a one-page handout for patients that lists the Web sites your physicians recommend;

- **Finding online patient support groups that you would recommend** — these support groups are flourishing on the Internet and communication with other patients with the same medical condition can really help patients;

- **Developing policies and procedures about how patients can access your practice via the Internet.** Look online or through your specialty society for services that help medical groups develop custom Web sites – some services allow patients to develop their own private Web pages and even will report lab results; and

- **Developing clear parameters if you wish to have patients e-mail you.** For example, will you accept urgent requests via e-mail? How swiftly can you commit to responding to e-mail inquiries? Can patients schedule appointments via e-mail?

If you use e-mail or the Web to communicate private information to patients, make sure to implement encryption strategies in compliance with HIPAA.

Patients who use the Internet can help your practice same time and money. Here how it works: patients who go online and find good information learn more about their medical conditions. This knowledge can make them more likely to comply with physician-recommended treatments. Better compliance can help speed recovery and reduce the volume of clinical questions, which often come in by telephone. This self-knowledge promotes more responsibility and patients rely less on what, at times, seems like constant communication with your practice.

Guide your employees' Internet use

Concerned about giving your staff Internet access? Many practices worry about staff spending too much time surfing or shopping online. Yes, abusing Web access privileges is possible, but the demands of most staff jobs are so significant that most people can find few spare moments for online foolishness. If you think that e-mail or Internet access will help patients or will help the office improve its productivity, then don't let fears of Web abuse stand in the way. That said, establish a clear policy for personal use of the Internet while at work.

Sample Internet use policy:

Because of the business implications and potential for misunderstandings as to employee conduct, no employee may use the practice's computers for his/her personal use unless the employee's supervisor grants approval. This includes accessing the Internet, playing computer games or using e-mail. The policy is in force at all times: before work, during work hours, after work or during lunch or breaks. Even if approved by your supervisor, personal use of the Internet should be infrequent, of short duration and may not interfere with work duties. The Practice may monitor, measure and track the use and performance of its systems for

245

technical or other reasons at any time, and may access any information contained in its systems.

To avoid any personal use, utilize readily available software to lock users into only Web sites that you designate.

Document management

Document management systems offer a wide variety of automation options for medical practice operations. Use these systems to store and retrieve information from documents electronically. Electronic storage and retrieval of documents also can create a "quasi" electronic medical record.

Here are some ways that your practices can use document management:

- Take your transcribed office notes – if you receive them in an electronic format such as a Word document – and organize them by patient identifiers. Using a database program, you can put the notes on a local area network (LAN). Each note will be accessible to the physicians who have passwords to use your internal network. This is a great solution for physicians who are on call and wish to review notes of a patient's recent office visits.

- Scan every piece of paper that comes into your office, from lab results to operative notes. Add the scanned images to the document management database (described above). Scanning explanation of benefits will help improve efficiency in the billing office (no more searching for EOBs to submit claims for secondary insurance).

- Use eFax (www.efax.com) or similar tools to translate all incoming faxes directly into electronic files for easy filing and retreival. Use patient identifiers to store faxed lab results, radiology reports, nursing home patient status updates and more.

- Use business card scanning software (such as www.bizcard reader.com) to scan vendor and other business contact information into an electronic database that all staff can access whenever they need to call for supplies, repairs or services.

- Scan patients' insurance cards and driver's licenses at registration. Automated systems like www. medicscan.com transfer the image to an electronic file that can be imported and attached to the patient's account.

Picture archiving and communication systems or PACS are more sophisticated – and more expensive – types of document management system. Many radiology practices use PACS because the radiological images that they must store and retrieve contain a massive amount of digital information – far more than a mere word processing document system could hold. As the cost of PACS comes down, expect more practices – maybe yours – to take advantage of these powerful new storage systems.

Document management saves money

Have you looked at the cost of storing the hundreds – maybe even thousands – of old records that you must maintain to comply with record retention laws? Some medical practices are beating the high cost of document storage by using CD-ROMs to hold thousands of scanned document images. You'll need a high-speed scanner and some staff time, but the reduction in storage fees often pays for the scanner within the first 12 months. Instead of stressing our your existing staff, save money by hiring high school and college students to do the scanning after hours or in a back room.

If you do scan old records – check your state records retention laws for how long you need to keep records – make several copies of each CD-ROM. Store them in several different secure locations in case of an emergency.

Personal digital assistants

Personal digital assistants (PDAs) became popular in the 1990s, and can now be found in the pocket of many physicians. Although some are just for personal use, PDAs can offer a host of opportunities to automate certain functions to improve efficiency:

Charge capture. Encourage physicians to use their PDAs to capture charges, particularly in the hospital, nursing home and other non-office locations. If you don't capture all those charges, it means you don't get paid for them. Place PDA docking stations where physicians can quickly download the charge information when they return to the office from the surgery or after hospital rounds. Some charge capture software interfaces with the practice management system through a wireless connection, thus allowing you to ditch the docking station. Remember, however, that someone must key the charges into the PDA in the first place. If you have a physician who never remembers to record charges on old-fashioned index cards, then don't expect the PDA to magically solve this forgetfulness.

Address book. Use as an address book for referring physicians. Send them office notes, hospital discharge summaries or operative reports by routing the documents through an online connection in your PDA directly to their fax numbers or e-mail accounts. Only route documents if the communication is secure.

Calendars. Keep everything from the physician's operating room schedule to medical staff meetings on the PDA. Physicians can keep their personal schedules on the same PDA, too.

Prescriptions. PDAs can help the prescription process in several ways. A PDA-based prescription system can help physicians keep track of which drugs are on which formulary and reduce the number of calls from pharmacists suggesting substitutions. It also provides appropriate dosing and contraindications. Best of all, these systems allow physicians to send electronic prescriptions directly to the pharmacy – no more calls from patients who lost their paper scrip or pharmacists who can't interpret the physicians' handwriting.

Coding and documentation. Accurate coding and documentation are critical to get paid appropriately. PDA-based coding software offers coding guidance, note templates and more.

Reference. Reference materials, such as Harrison's Textbook of Medicine and Physician's Desk Reference, are only two of the many useful resources available for use with some PDAs. Even better, these texts can be queried through key word searches to help you find what you need more efficiently.

Knowledge. Database tools such as www.medicalinforetreiver. com can help when the physician is on call in the middle of the night and can't access professional assistance from colleagues. These tools support clinical decision-making and can access a host of resources. Those who use PDAs with Internet connections can find services that abstract pertinent medical literature.

Point of Care. Choose from dozens of point-of-care medical calculators, algorithms, and checkers designed for PDA users. For example, PregCalc is at www.thenar.com/pregcalc.

Call schedules. Keep call schedules on everyone's PDA so you can eliminate the ubiquitous "master calendar" that physicians and clinical staff have to stop by the office to look at, or call an already busy staff member to check.

Today's PDAs can combine telephone, messaging, e-mail, video images, Internet connections and other functions in one device. So, trade in your pager, phone, e-mail account, fax, voicemail and even your computer for a single, all-purpose hand-held PDA.

E-Prescribing and malpractice discounts

E-prescribing means using technology – usually software on a handheld device – to decide on the right medication, look for interactions and allergies, check the medication choice against a formulary and then electronically send a prescription to a pharmacy. Because e-prescribing enhances patient safety, some malpractice carriers offer premium discounts to physicians who use e-prescribing. Check with your insurer.

Electronic medical records

"Electronic medical records" is a term that means taking everything that is contained on paper in a patient's medical record and automating it. But it's more than just getting rid of the paper and automating the information. Practices that have found the most success with EMRs are those that use their systems to get information to users faster and with less hassle.

...you need an EMR when...

- Your practice's multiple sites are close enough in proximity that patients go to either facility and your staff must spend hours each day pulling patient charts and faxing them between sites.

- You pack up a rolling suitcase with patient charts each morning for a staff member to drive to a satellite clinic for that day's appointments. When an additional patient walks in, staff at your central facility must break from other duties to find and fax the walk-in patient's charts to the satellite.

- Your practice does not respond to its large volume of triage calls for hours because the messages are recorded and callbacks must wait until the patients' charts are found. Many hours of staff time are wasted taking and routing messages, as well as pulling and filing charts needed for them.

- Charts that your physicians need for prescription refills or to answer triage questions are often found at the bottom of stack on the desk of the physician who is notoriously behind on dictation.

- The billing office's appeal of an insurer's claims denial is delayed several days until, finally, the patient's chart is located on someone's desk. In it is the documentation that can support the appeal for payment.

- The administrator has to go to the office on Saturday afternoon to let in the physician who is on weekend call so he can find the chart of a patient who is being admitted to the hospital.

- A physician must be paged at home because the colleague covering his calls that day cannot read his illegible handwritten note of the patient's last office visit – or the treating physician just makes a guess.

- Despite your best efforts, many of the hundreds of patient telephone calls your practice's triage nurses and staff receive each day are never charted.

- A physician receives a call from an out-of-state ER where one of her patients was injured while on vacation and the ER physician needs the patient's records quickly.

- A physician realizes months later that he never received or saw the results of a patient's biopsy that he ordered.

- Drug recalls require countless hours of staff time pouring over paper records to determine which patients should be contacted regarding their medication.

An EMR can resolve all of these problems – and more!

Although it's not an all-inclusive list, here are the benefits of an EMR for your practice:

- Integrates national standards of care;

- Puts updated, complete and legible information about the patient in the physician's hands at the point of care;

- Delivers and monitors health maintenance initiatives;

- Stamps signatures, as well as times and dates, electronically;

- Facilitates correspondence with referring physicians;

- Evaluates office workflow by monitoring patients from registration to checkout;

- Avoids the cost of paper and other charting supplies;

- Decreases space and potentially staffing needs related to medical records and transcription;

- Accesses up-to-date information on a real-time basis at the office, satellite clinic, home, hospital or elsewhere;

- Improves physician's ability to manage care while on call because information is accessible;

- Identifies candidates for treatment based on new clinical guidelines;

- Facilitates drug recalls;

- Enhances compliance with privacy regulations by restricting access to designated users only;

- Reviews candidates and monitor participants in clinical trials;

- Allows multiple users to access records simultaneously from separate locations;

- Records telephone, e-mail and other non-face-to-face communication seamlessly;

- Identifies and monitors coding patterns;

- Interfaces multiple clinical and administrative systems;

- Improves ability to document all services and code appropriately for them;

- Documents and queries orders, medications, allergies, etc., with ease;

- Transmits patient records to remote providers in an emergency; and

- Monitors tests ordered and prompts for missing results.

An EMR can streamline your practice into a more efficient office. However, it's not enough to have an EMR – you need to make it work for you. If your practice still takes phone messages on pieces of paper which then float around the office and get lost or if you still print patient records from your EMR and drag them in a suitcase to the satellite clinic, then your EMR isn't doing you any good. To be successful, an EMR should eliminate duplication and streamline workflow.

Before you sign a purchase contract, consider these tips about your purchase:

- Get the vendor's commitment to provide several days of staff training, as well as to train a staff member or physician to monitor and fix routine issues.

- Make sure that the vendor updates the system's medication information and clinical content modules at least quarterly.

- Ask if the system features templates that are specific to your physicians' – and their specialty – needs.

- Be careful about buying an EMR that has no track record of smoothly interfacing with your practice management software; alternatively, the EMR (equipped with the necessary administrative functionality) could replace your practice management system.

- Make sure you know all the new hardware and equipment interfaces or upgrades that you must purchase to make the EMR work.

- Negotiate the terms of service agreements before purchase.

- Estimate the drop in productivity, and if necessary, the financial impact of it.

- Plan for the system to go down – and ask the vendor to commit to helping you establish a back-up plan.

EMR costs vary tremendously, prices are dropping and system capabilities are expanding. That said, larger practices still seem to negotiate the best deals. But the days in which EMR was marketed only to large practices are gone. Smaller-sized practices, as well as larger ones, have more options than systems based on client-server technology. Application service providers or Web-based application models can keep purchase and startup costs low.

Preparing your practice

Use careful judgment when it comes to adopting any technology, whether it's for patients, physicians, or staff. Practices often read about a new piece of technology, and introduce it without considering the effect on workflow. Technology can significantly change processes; if you're not prepared for this or haven't thought it through, disaster can result.

When you consider a piece of technology, planning is in order. Even if the technology looks great, consider how it will work on a day-to-day basis in your practice. Gather a workgroup of everyone, or at least representatives from several departments, who will be affected by the technology. Then, create two flow charts: one showing the workflow as it exists today and another one showing how it will change with the new technology. What are the implications for your physicians, your staff, your facility and your patients?

Don't overlook even the simplest of things: A physician who has never learned to type will have trouble keeping up with his patient load if he must suddenly switch to an electronic medical record that requires use of a keyboard. Will you give him typing lessons? How long will it take him to peck at the keyboard? Will you hire a scribe for him? Will you allow him to continue to dictate?

Physician productivity could decline over the short-term while a new system is implemented. To minimize that impact, develop templates, pull-down menus and other features that will mesh your physicians' work styles with the system's requirements. Contract for on-site support to fix glitches or respond to users about problems immediately. A day of on-site support won't do; contract for several weeks, if not more.

Conduct a financial proforma. It doesn't need to be anything fancy, but make sure that you measure what the technology costs (including service) and what you will gain. The benefits may include more direct revenue, reduced cost or simply better customer service. The point is to know exactly what you're getting into so there won't be any surprises.

Deciding on a vendor is difficult. Since every practice is different, you can only rely on yourself. That is, just because a vendor works for a practice next door, doesn't mean it will work for you. Do your own homework.

After you've decided on the technology and the vendor — train, train, and re-train. Don't assume anything. People are often embarrassed to admit that they're technologically challenged, so start from the beginning. As you hire more staff and physicians who have grown up with the information superhighway, the basic training won't be a necessity. Until then, make sure you allow everyone to start at a basic level.

Seven easy ways to make a technology purchase

In a busy practice with little time to spare for thoughtful evaluation, it's easy — and expensive — to make a bad technology purchase. Use this advice before you buy.

1. Don't just fall in love with the new technology's bells and whistles. Do this and you could end up with a system that does a great job of solving problems you never had while creating many new ones. Instead, buy technology that will improve your margins and expand your capacity. Buy technology that will help you manage your operations more efficiently and effectively. Buy technology that will get the job done.

2. Don't forget about your people and processes. Practices that make this error are the ones that buy systems that require a busy physician to hunt through multiple screens for patient information during the visit. Instead, keep in mind that the software you buy will affect the way your practice works and even the way your physicians practice. Know your patient flow processes inside and out before making a purchase. Know before you buy if your physicians are comfortable typing, pointing and clicking, or using a voice-automated program.

3. Don't give everyone – or your vendor – ownership of the project. Expecting that your vendor will handle all implementation concerns or that problems can somehow resolve by themselves is asking for trouble. Make sure that one internal person takes leadership on the project and can make the day-to-day decisions that will inevitably come up. Rely on this person for troubleshooting and advice for related software purchases.

4. Don't ignore your infrastructure. Ignore infrastructure details before you buy and you may end up buying new hardware. Of course, your operating system is critical, but don't forget to also assess your current system's processors, memory and disk space. Read the software vendor's "minimum technical requirements" to find out if your computer, networking and other software programs are compatible with and capable of handling the new technology.

5. Don't give the vendor control over your buying process. If you don't define what you want out of the new system, then the vendor will. Instead, figure out what you are trying to accomplish by buying the new system. List the capabilities you expect from the system before you start interviewing vendors.

6. Don't evaluate vendors only on technical capabilities. Instead, ask vendors if they provide customer support during your working hours. Ask them if ongoing training is available. Have they dealt with physician practices of your specialty before? Is their software installation and customer service handled by their staff or by contractors? How long will it really take to get the system working? Is there an extra charge for support, training and implementation? What happens when the system goes down?

7. Don't forget to ask for references. Software is a complex purchase. Buying software like an EMR is the beginning of a partnership with your vendor. It's in your best interests to ask vendors of any major technology to give you the names of several references. Be sure to ask for references that medical practice of similar size and the specialty or specialty mix as yours. Supplement the vendor's list by calling around to colleagues at other practices, and hop on a practice management listserv to ask for feedback about the system.

Tap into a great resource

If you are interested in integrating technology into your practice, but don't think you can afford it and can't do it yourself, consider calling your local community college or university to find someone who can assist you with the project and even do some custom programming for you. Give them your ideas, and see what they can do. It's a cost-effective way to get the job done.

Use technology to get results

If you just want to integrate technology in a limited fashion in your practice, or supplement your high-tech office with some additional automation, try some of these ideas.

- Use e-mail to redistribute telephone and other incoming messages. Set up accounts with names like triagenurse @yourpractice.com or billing@yourpractice.com to help users direct their messages. The traffic that comes into these e-mail boxes will help you track where the messages go and what people ask about.

- Sign all of your staff and physicians onto instant messaging through an online service. Instant messaging works well for everything from reminders about staff meetings to announcing the arrival of patients for their appointments.

- Use online calendars (e.g., Microsoft Outlook calendar) to manage waiting lists of patients, tickler files for everything from insurance appeals to lab results, staff events and others.

- Send patients their billing statements via e-mail. As part of your privacy policy, include a check off box next to the patient's email address that gives permission to send "e-statements." Link them to your Web site, and allow them to pay their bill online.

- Use electronic time clocks that allow staff to clock in and out at their workstations each day. Times are monitored, and downloaded to a payroll system where checks can be printed automatically.

- Offer a Web site that patients can access for information about your practice, as well as to request referrals, appointments, refills, lab results and account balances.

- Network with other practices through chat rooms or e-mail listservs offered by your professional association, specialty society and state or local medical societies.

- Sign up for a coding advice service so that you can e-mail tough coding questions to a coding expert – and get accurate answers fast.

- Access the products and services of professional organizations like the Medical Group Management Association (MGMA).

- Look for the current clinical findings and management research through Internet search engines such as www.google.com or www.pubmed.gov.

- Buy medical and office supplies, equipment, furniture and other office necessities.

- Save time and money on continuing medical education (CME) by taking classes or finding CME-accredited articles online instead of attending on-site conferences.

- Participate in Web casts for CME, management and staff training.

- Take advantage of online insurance coverage and benefits eligibility verification, as well as claims status inquiry services that many insurance companies offer online through direct access or portals like www.medunite.com.

- Try interactive voice response (IVR) software to help manage patient collections.

- Use direct claims submission if your insurance companies offer it. Post charges and – voila – transmit them directly to the insurance company via the Web for faster payment.

- Utilize electronic payment posting and funds transfer to eliminate manual posting staff and get your money in the door faster.

- Use fun sites like www.epraise.com and www.hrtools.com to help manage employees and to boost morale.

- Buy gift certificates for employee rewards from thousands of retail establishments.

- Manage documents better through services like www.efax.com, which transforms incoming faxes into e-mail messages. Lab reports and the like can be easier to store and locate when they are in a digital format.

- Get free reminder e-mails about important dates, like employees' birthdays and employment anniversaries using Web sites like www.hallmarkreminder.com or www.birthday alarm.com.

- Post your employee schedule, policy manual, managed-care manual, call schedule, hospital rounds list, and other pertinent information on a secure Web site so you or your staff can access it quickly.

- Manage your credentialing online.

- Utilize online bill payment services to save on postage and increase the efficiency of your accounts payable process.

- Access online interpretation services if a non-English speaking patient presents to the office without an interpreter.

- Throw away the little dictation tapes, and utilize digital transcription. Transmit transcription files online to vendors who can turnaround your dictation faster and cheaper.

- Establish online connections to your practice management system and electronic medical record for employees working in functions conducive to off-site work.

- Use a digital camera to take pictures of patients – or their physical conditions. Use photos to identify patients by sight instead of just name, store pre- and post-procedure photographs, or paste photographic images in correspondence to referring physicians.

- Give your patients identification cards with barcodes. Allow patients to "register" with their identification cards when they enter your facility.

- Utilize a tablet PC to deliver patient education in the exam room or take hand-written chart notes electronically that can be integrated into your practice's records system.

- Barcode order forms, lab vials, paper charts or other items that need to be tracked.

Conclusion: It pays to be creative in your use of technology. Technology can improve your efficiency and reduce costs.

New generation of users

As new, technology-dependent physicians and employees enter the workforce, integrating technology into your practice won't just be fun and games – it will be essential. There are so many ways to integrate automation into your practice; it only takes a creative mind, and some careful planning to harness technology to work for you.

Chapter 10

FUNDAMENTAL FINANCIALS

Key Chapter Lessons

> Identify key financial concepts

> Learn about fixed and variable costs

> Calculate your overhead rate

> Analyze your break-even point

> Understand how expense reduction can backfire

Advanced Concept

> 25 strategies to cut costs

Key financial concepts

Contribution margin: The revenue generated by an additional volume of services minus the variable costs to produce the volume equals the "contribution margin." For example, an in-house lab generates $20,000 in revenue and incurs $5,000 in variable expenses to perform an additional number of tests. Thus, the lab has produced a contribution margin of $15,000 to help cover fixed expenses. In general, when the contribution margin is positive, performing additional services is a good financial decision.

Fixed cost: An expense that remains the same without regard to change in volume.

Leverage: The ability to use a resource to increase the value of an asset. For example, leveraging a physician's time by having a nurse return a portion of the calls allows the physician to spend more time with that day's patients. While the nurse answers the telephone calls, the physician can generate more revenue by seeing the next patient. *(This definition simplifies the twin issues of operating and financial leverage. Operating leverage refers to the extent a business commits itself to higher levels of fixed costs. Financial leverage refers to the extent to which a business gets its cash resources from debt as opposed to equity.)*

Overhead rate: Operating expenses divided by revenue.

Provider: Anyone who can bill third-party payers for services (generally, physicians and midlevel providers).

Variable cost: An expense that changes in direct relationship to change in an activity associated with the generation of revenue. For instance, each time a physician sees a patient, a quantity of medical supplies is used. Thus, medical supply costs vary directly (up or down) with the number of patients seen.

Volume: The number of patients the practice's providers handle.

The fundamental financials

When patient flow runs smoothly, a practice's revenue (cash flow) and physician productivity improve. So, now that I have presented the details of patient flow, let's look at what can happen — financially — when you improve it.

When you subtract the practice's operating costs from the total revenue collected by the practice, the result is net operating income. Practices owned by physicians call this net income — physician income or physician compensation. A practice that has other types of owners, such as a hospital or a physician management company, might just call this net operating income: income.

No matter what the ownership structure is, achieving a positive net operating income is critical to sustained financial performance. By increasing your revenue and/or reducing your expenses, your practice can increase operating income. This chapter focuses on costs and how to leverage them to increase your income.

Controlling cost is at the heart of running operations more smoothly and more profitably in any type of business. Costs (called expenses when costs are incurred to generate revenues) measure the use of the resources, or assets, that the practice uses to produce revenue. Resources that your practice uses everyday to bring in revenue will likely include clinical and non-clinical staff, equipment, supplies and the facility.

An often-quoted statistic is your overhead rate, which is a measure of your practice's ability to use non-revenue-producing (operating) expenses to leverage its revenue-producing expenses (physicians and midlevel providers). The overhead rate is determined by dividing your operating expenses by your revenue.

In this chapter, I will examine how the operating and staff resources of the practice are used to leverage physicians' (or any billable providers') time to produce revenue.

Fixed cost: Get to know it and how to measure it

There are two broad categories of costs: fixed and variable. Let's first focus on fixed costs – expenses that remain stable regardless of volume.

Fixed costs can include:

- Support staff, wages and benefits
- Information services (computer and telecommunications)
- Furniture and equipment
- Building and occupancy (utilities, housekeeping, grounds, etc.)
- Professional liability and other insurance premiums
- Promotion and marketing
- Miscellaneous operating costs (e.g., administrative services) that do not depend on patient volume

These fixed costs do not vary with the volume of patients. That is, if your practice sees 20 patients on Monday and 19 on Tuesday, your practice doesn't pay 1/20th less on Tuesday for its rent, telephones, support staff, liability insurance and so on.

A subdivision of fixed cost is step-fixed cost. This represents the costs that remain fixed until the volume of whatever activity they are supporting increases or decreases significantly; then the cost of that activity – the resources it uses – adjusts up or down accordingly. An example of a step-fixed cost would be the cost of hiring an additional medical assistant to help the practice handle higher volume when it increases from 15 patients a day to 30 patients a day.

Here are two important things to remember about fixed and step-fixed costs:

1. Fixed and step-fixed costs do not change because of minor fluctuations in the volume of services provided or in the number of patients seen. That is, if your patient volume increases from an average of 18 per day to 19 per day, you won't run out to hire another medical assistant.

2. Fixed and step-fixed costs together account for more than 85 percent of the total operating cost structure in most medical practices. (We'll look at the other 15 percent – variable costs – in the next section of this chapter.)

Specialties with high variable costs

Some medical practices have higher variable costs than others do. In an oncology practice, chemotherapy alone can represent 15 percent of the practice's total operating cost. Because chemotherapy is utilized on a per patient basis, it is considered a variable cost.

Variable costs

Although the majority of your expenses are fixed, or stable, without regard to volume, you will have certain other expenses that occur only when your practice provides a service. These are the variable costs.

A variable cost is an expense that goes up and down in relation to fluctuations in the activity that caused the cost to occur in the first place. The activity, or resource consumption, that causes most of the variable costs that occur in most medical practices is physicians seeing patients. That is, if a physician did not see a patient, these costs would not occur.

To see what generally makes up a variable cost, let's assume the service being provided is a patient visit. When a patient walks in your door, your practice will generate paperwork, including an encounter form. The patient is given a gown to dress for the visit. Certain medical supplies may be used during the visit. After the patient leaves, a claim is generated, which is followed by one or more patient statements. All of these items – paperwork, gown, medical supplies, claims and billing statements – are expenses that occurred solely because of that patient's visit. These are variable costs.

Unlike fixed costs (rent, computer system, medical assistant, etc.), if the patient cancels the visit, you do not incur the cost of consuming the resources included in the variable cost category.

Using total practice cost

Your overhead rate describes the resources your practice must use to generate revenue. The higher the rate, the less there is to contribute to physician income. Your overhead rate will largely depend on your specialty. In surgical specialties it may be as low as 30 percent, while in primary care overhead can be as high as 60 percent.

Surgical specialties have the benefit of utilizing the hospital's resources (operating room nurses, registered nurses in the hospital) with relatively small office staff while primary care groups bear all of the costs of an office, typically seeing patients five days per week. Although surgical specialties still have receptionists, billers, telephone operators, etc., they have proportionately lower costs than their office-based colleagues. However, the percent of total costs for any practitioner, regardless of specialty, is typically 50 percent personnel expenses and 50 percent operating expenses. That is, out of $100,000 in total practice costs (exclusive of the provider's compensation), $50,000 is spent on personnel and $50,000 on operating expenses. In addition, as described later, since the overhead rate is a ratio of costs to revenue, if revenue (the denominator) is higher, than the rate falls. Therefore, because surgical specialties have lower operating costs and higher revenue than other physicians, their overhead rates are lower.

What's your "Total Practice Cost"?

List your practice's costs on an annual basis.

Your annual fixed costs

$_____ Support staff wages and benefits (medical, vacation, sick leave, retirement contribution, employer's FICA contribution, etc.)

$_____ Information services (computer and telecommunications)

$_____ Furniture and equipment

$_____ Building and occupancy (utilities, housekeeping, grounds, etc.)

$_____ Professional liability and other insurance premiums

$_____ Promotion and marketing

$_____ Other miscellaneous operating costs that do not depend on patient volume

= $_____ total fixed costs

Your annual variable costs

$_____ Administrative supplies and services

$_____ Medical supplies and drugs

$_____ Laundry and linen

$_____ Other miscellaneous operating costs that depend on patient volume

= $_____ Total variable costs

total fixed costs + total variable costs = total practice costs

GETTING STARTED

Variable costs to track

❑ Administrative supplies and services

❑ Medical supplies and drugs

❑ Laundry and linen

❑ Miscellaneous operating costs (lab supplies, chemotherapy, etc.) that depend on patient volume)

Once you've completed the "What's your total practice cost?" worksheet, it is a simple step to determine your overhead rate. To compute your overhead rate, you will also need to know your practice's total annual practice revenue (unless you choose to calculate this on a quarterly basis, in which case you would divide quarterly operating cost by quarterly revenue). Divide total annual practice costs by the total annual practice revenue from the worksheet (include both fixed and variable costs) and the result is the overhead rate, which is expressed as a percentage.

[total practice costs (fixed + variable) / total practice revenue] * 100 = overhead rate

Since the majority of a practice's costs are fixed, or stable, almost regardless of volume, it is critical to determine the level of volume your practice must handle to cover its fixed costs. The revenue brought in from any volume achieved after this break-even point (and after variable costs are subtracted) is profit. Profit adds to the net operating income that is critical to the practice's financial success.

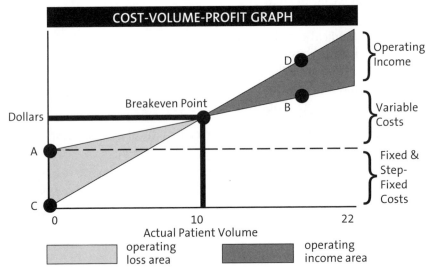

A = Fixed Costs + Step Fixed Costs
  Fixed Costs and Step Fixed Costs include rent, staff, utilities, malpractice insurance, information systems, furniture/equipment.
B = Total Costs (Variable + Fixed) at 20 patients per day
  Variable costs include administrative supplies, medical supplies, drugs.
C = Revenue at 0 patients seen.
D = Revenue at 20 patients per day.
The CVP Graph describes the relationship between cost, volume and profit in a medical practice.

Overhead rate

> The overhead rate equals all those costs that are used to support the providers in a practice to generate revenue. These expenses do not include the physician's income or benefits or midlevel providers' income and benefits. The rate captures the practice's ability to turn operating costs (the numerator) into revenue (the denominator).

Once you calculate your overhead rate, you will know how many dollars are being expended on operating costs per dollar earned. For example, Family Practice Associates calculated its operating costs at $456,955 and its revenue at $985,001. Using the formula, the overhead rate is 46.39 percent. For every dollar earned or collected by the practice, $0.46 is spent on overhead costs.

We would presume that the majority (if not all) of the remainder ($0.54) is consumed by the physician(s) as income. The goal is to have as low an overhead rate as possible (that is, you would rather spend $0.40 on operating costs for each dollar collected than $0.50, as that would leave more money to distribute as income); however, you want to remember that this is a ratio of costs to revenue. Therefore, you can't just focus on cost reduction because by doing so, you may simply reduce revenue, thereby leaving the overhead rate unchanged, or worse, even higher.

Don't just focus on cost-cutting opportunities when trying to reduce your overhead rate. Increased revenue also affects the overhead rate. Later on, I'll discuss the key role your providers play in increasing revenue.

Decreasing Overhead the Wrong Way

Family Practice Associates (FPA) was disappointed at its overhead rate of 46.39 percent. They decided to take action by leasing out three of its exam rooms to a urologist in the suite next door who needed extra space. Therefore, FPA reduced its lease expense by $4,900, which dropped its operating expenses to $452,055. However, the loss of the exam rooms also reduced the volume of patients that FPA was able to see by two percent. Because the physicians only had two and one-half exam rooms from which to work, FPA's revenue declined by $19,700 to $965,301.

Recalculating its overhead rate, FPA divided its new expenses of $452,055 by its new revenue of $965,301. With this cost-cutting method, its new overhead rate actually increased to 46.83 percent. FPA failed to recognize that its overhead rate consists of costs and revenue. Simply reducing its costs was not the answer to reducing its overhead rate, particularly because it actually decreased its revenue, thus increasing its overhead rate.

What's your volume/cost break-even point?

At some point during the average month, your practice will handle enough volume to break-even. But when? A practice needs to know whether this break-even point will occur earlier or later in the month, or if it will occur at all. The following exercise demonstrates how one practice was able to determine the number of patient visits needed to break-even in a typical month.

Let's assume the practice had one physician. Let's also assume that each visit the physician provided produced an average of $50 in revenue. Based on a review of a few previous months' invoices and other records, the variable cost (linen, administrative supplies and medical supplies used per visit) was calculated at $5 per visit. The $5 per visit is based on the total variable costs incurred during the months in review divided by the number of visits during that month. A quick glance at the practice's readily available records (office rent, insurance premiums, administrative staff salaries, equipment leases, etc.) showed that its total fixed cost was $10,000 a month. The physician sees 500 patients per month, and wants to know if this is adequate to break-even.

revenue per visit:	$50 per visit
total visits:	500
total revenue:	$25,000 ($50 * 500)
desired physician income:	$12,500/month (or $150,000/year)
fixed costs:	$10,000
variable costs:	$2,500 ($5 per visit * 500 visits)

To determine the volume of patients needed to break-even, we must observe the total costs that the physician would like to cover, which are the fixed costs plus the desired physician income, which together equal $22,500. Because some of the revenue per visit, which is $50, must be used for variable expenses, which are $5 per visit, we know that we can use $45 per visit to allocate toward the desired expense base. $45 is the contribution margin expressed on a unit of service basis. The $45 is referred to as "unit contribution margin" because it contributes to covering the practice's fixed costs. Therefore, we can divide the total fixed cost (including income target) of $22,500 by the $45 unit contribution margin, which equals 500 patient visits — the break-even volume.

We can see that 500 patient visits per month allow this practice to break-even; that is, cover the costs (physician and operating) incurred. With 500 patient visits per month, the physician covers current costs and receives $150,000 in annual income.

How many patients needed to support physician income?

Now, let's approach the break-even question from a different angle. Suppose you start out knowing that each of your physicians wants to earn $240,000 per year, and you know what it costs to run the practice. Your question is: how many patients do each of the practice's physicians need to see to achieve their desired $240,000 in annual income ($20,000 per month) per physician.

WORKSHEET
Visits needed to support income goal

What is the number of patient visits that your physician needs to meet his income goals?

patient visits: ?
fixed expenses: $10,000 per month
variable expenses: $5/visit

Assuming the physician wants to receive $240,000 in annual income, we know that we need to average $20,000 a month in physician income. We also know that the fixed expenses are $10,000 per month for a total of $120,000 per year. We also know that we are receiving $50 per visit, but we have to use $5 of that to pay for our variable expenses. Therefore, we have $45 left over for fixed expenses and physician income.

How many visits do we need per month? Divide the $30,000 in fixed costs and physician income by $45 and you arrive at 667 visits per month.

fixed cost ($10,000/month) + physician income ($20,000/month) = total fixed cost

revenue per visit ($50) – variable expense per visit ($5) = unit contribution margin per visit ($45)

fixed expense ($30,000/month) / unit contribution margin per visit ($45) = visits needed per month (667)

The Answer: If your physician wants an income of $240,000 per year, he needs to see 667 visits per month, or 8,000 per year.

WORKSHEET
What's your break-even point?

Use this worksheet to determine the number of patient visits your group needs to meet its physician income goals. To figure the break-even point for your own group, use the data you gathered in the "What's your total practice cost" worksheet. To complete this worksheet, you'll also need to know the level of income or physician compensation your physicians or practice owner(s) want to achieve. In the typical physician-owned medical practice, this income amount is called, "physician compensation." If you want to invest some of the revenues in the practice, such as for a new computer system, or a facility expansion, then determine the amount of investment to make.

Input your data (write in your practice's amounts in spaces provided and then transfer the amounts to the blanks according to the letter per category). For this analysis, use annual data for each category.

(a) desired physician income: _____

(b) fixed expenses: _____

(c) investment: _____

(d) variable expenses per visit: _____

(e) average revenue per visit: _____

fixed expense + investment + income = total fixed expense

(b)_____ + (c)_____ + (a)_____ =
(g)_____

average revenue per visit − variable cost per visit = unit contribution margin per visit

(e)_____ − (d)_____ = (h)_____

fixed cost / unit contribution margin per visit = visits needed per year

(g)_____ /(h)_____ = _____

Expenses: The bottom line

Intuitively, we know that the more patients a physician sees, the greater the revenue for the practice. We also know that per visit revenue can vary and that variable costs and step-fixed costs also increase as volume increases. But what if your physicians already work long hours and see as many patients as they feel they can handle? What if their revenue enhancement options are somewhat limited? What if they also want to maintain or, possibly, raise their income goals? Since most physicians – like most people – want to control how many hours they work and meet their income goals, reducing fixed costs can be a good route to increasing income or, at least, maintaining it when reimbursement rates are static or declining. Attacking fixed costs can be an especially advantageous strategy if your physicians are experiencing declining reimbursements or increased competition for patients and cannot easily expand into more profitable product lines.

If you can reduce your fixed cost base, you can reduce the number of visits your practice needs to break-even and achieve the physician's desired income.

Lowering fixed costs to break-even at lower volume

Here's one way to project the effect of a fixed cost reduction. The physician in this practice wanted to have a few more hours off each month for activities that did not bring in income, such as volunteering at a free clinic, attending CME classes or attending a child's school activities once in a while. How could this physician still achieve an income goal of $240,000 annually ($20,000 per month) and continue to break-even in the practice?

To reduce fixed costs, this physician plans to move from a facility that costs $2,000 a month in rent to one in the same neighborhood that costs $1,000 per month (50 percent reduction in occupancy expenses). This move would reduce the practice's fixed costs to $9,000 per month. However, before signing the lease on the new facility, the administrator wanted to determine what effect the fixed cost reduction would have on the number of patients the physician had to see each month to meet income goals. The practice currently receives an average of $50 per visit, which is not expected to change if the practice decides to move.

Pre-move
fixed costs: $10,000 per month
physician income: $20,000 per month
variable expenses: $5 per visit
patient visits: 667 per month

Post-move
fixed expenses: $9,000 per month
physician income: $20,000 per month
variable expenses: $5 per visit
patient visits: _____?

With the reduced rental expense, the practice now had $9,000 per month in fixed costs plus the $20,000 the physician wanted to earn, for a total of $29,000 in monthly fixed expenses. We know that the practice received $50 per visit, but had to use $5 to pay the variable expenses for each visit. That left the practice with $45 to pay its fixed expenses per visit (unit contribution margin), plus what the physician wanted to receive in income. So, how many fewer patient visits can the physician see per month to continue achieving those goals at the lower rent?

We can determine the number of patient visits needed per month to meet fixed expenses by dividing fixed expense per month ($29,000) by unit contribution margin per visit ($45) to get 644 patient visits per month.

**[fixed expense per month ($9,000)
+ physician income ($20,000)] /
unit contribution margin per visit ($45)
= 644 patient visits per month**

By reducing the fixed costs by $1,000, the physician could see 22 fewer patients a month, and still achieve the desired annual income of $240,000. The exact number of hours freed up would depend on the time per visit.

Be careful about expense reductions. Expenses that improve the physician's productivity are well worth it. Attempts to slash fixed costs will backfire if they end up causing great inconvenience to patients, reduce physician and staff productivity or, worse, reduce the quality of care or range of profitable services that your practice can provide. That's why many medical practices are embracing the concept of combining judicious fixed cost cuts with efforts to improve their patient flow processes.

An understanding of the fundamental financials, combined with a solid comprehension of patient flow opportunities, will allow you to implement operations changes in a cost-effective manner.

ADVANCED CONCEPT

25 ways to cut costs

Evaluate these 25 proven methods to cut costs in your practice:

1. **Reduce lease or rent payments** by moving, reducing workspace and/or renegotiating your current lease(s). If your leased your office space when the real estate market of office space was booming, you may be able to get a much better deal now.

2. **Reduce support staff expenses** by reevaluating staff positions and duties. Maybe improved processes and automation mean that some staff positions can be combined or eliminated without any loss in overall productivity? Could an employee with lower skills (and a lower wage) be able to handle certain functions?

3. **Evaluate your vendor contracts annually**, including those for medical and office supplies and equipment. Check competitors' prices and consider switching vendors. Don't forget about the smaller contracts, like those with your collection agency or electronic claims transmission carrier. Review service contracts every year to make sure that you're not paying for services that you don't need – or if you're paying high hourly rates when you could have a cheaper capitated service plan.

4. **Watch out for vendors that are increasing prices due to regulatory compliance** (e.g., transcription services that are hiking their rates because of HIPAA). Shop around for better pricing before you agree to pay their increased rates.

5. **Evaluate vendor value.** Don't just price shop – make sure that you are getting what you pay for. Did a vendor "adjust" a fee or add a service charge without telling you? Has the quality or timeliness of their service dropped?

6. **Review telecommunications costs,** including local and long distance telephone carriers. Carefully review bills to make sure you're not paying for services (like extra telephone lines or services) that you didn't ask for. Do the physicians need the cellular telephone plans' 1,000 "free" minutes-a-month, or is there a lower costing plan? Are you paying more than seven cents a minute for long distance? Is there a vendor who will bundle your Internet connection, long distance, cellular phone services or other services for a reduced fee? Do you have the best available rate for cell phones and pagers?

7. **Reduce the expenses allocated to your information system** – or at least free up money to be used for other technology improvements – by moving to an application service provider model for registration, scheduling and billing.

8. **Scrutinize your employee benefits structure** as well as the service of the benefits agent with whom you work. Can you pass along health care insurance cost increases to employees? Survey employees to see what benefits they value the most.

9. **Consider different options to reduce the impact of malpractice liability insurance premium hikes.** Can you change deductibles? Ask your malpractice insurance carrier if it offers a discount if physicians take risk management courses. What if you use an electronic medical record or

computerize prescriptions? Is your practice large enough to self-insure?

10. **Look for free continuing medical education (CME) on the Internet or in journals.** Consider low-cost, no travel options like audio conferences if travel expenses are eating away at your CME budget.

11. **Think about outsourcing billing, transcription, and even some front desk operations.** Every few years, reassess whether handling these processes in-house or outsourcing them is cheaper. Consider the vendor's performance before an outsourcing decision.

12. **Utilize scanning and digital imaging** to capture and store documents from patients' pictures to insurance cards. Reduce storage costs, paper supplies and copier equipment and service costs.

13. **Keep up with technology trends.** Would an automated reminder system save staff costs? What about automated referral processing? Automated charge entry? Automated lab results system?

14. **Evaluate your overtime costs monthly.** If you often pay for overtime, you may need to hire or reorganize. If you often pay billers overtime at the end of each month to catch up on claims filings, stop batching those claims and ask providers to submit claims at the end of every day. It will improve cash flow and eliminate overtime.

15. **Do a better job of retaining staff.** Hiring, training, and lost productivity costs make replacing an employee cost you three to six months of that employee's salary. High turnover costs money. Make sure your orientation and training processes, workload and office culture help keep employees around, not drive them off.

16. **Decrease statement mailings.** More practices mail no more than three patient statements – instead of six or eight – before taking other action. Cutting mailings in half saves more than $1.50 per patient, which will make a big difference over time. Do a better job of collecting payments at the time of service and you can eliminate most statement mailings.

17. **Cut out the middleman.** For example, submit claims directly to insurance carriers – or their Internet portals – at no cost instead of sending everything through a clearinghouse. Even though a clearinghouse may charge only a few pennies per claim, those pennies quickly become big bucks in today's busy practices.

18. **Dig for bargains.** Need medical or office equipment for your practice? Try shopping at www.ebay.com, other bargain Web sites or a used equipment store. Keep on the alert for a local business that is closing its doors and selling its furniture and equipment. Maybe another practice in your community is shutting its doors or consolidating. "Retro" is all the rage in interior design, and a quick paint job on old furniture and equipment will bring accolades from patients. Buying used can save you thousands.

19. **Track expenses.** Introduce an inventory system to track all expenses, even "little" things like toilet paper. Keep tabs on volume and price of what you use so you can comparison shop. You may discover, for example, that it's well worth it to join a membership discount club, like Sam's Club or Costco, and stock up on printer paper and paper towels four times a year, instead of paying top dollar for these items through your current supplier who delivers these items to your door.

20. **Give employees rewards that come from the heart, not just the checkbook.** Instead of a nominal annual cash bonus, consider giving time off with pay as an alternative reward. It costs you nothing as long as you don't have to bring in a replacement. In these time-starved days,

employees may actually prefer a little free time to a small cash reward.

21. **Assess your professional advisers.** Are you paying a retainer to anyone whose service you do not use or rarely use? What about bringing back in-house certain outsourced duties, such as bookkeeping? Is there a bright and eager person on staff who would happily take over bookkeeping duties in exchange for a small promotion?

22. **Explore exemptions.** If the expense of a managed-care or referral clerk is bogging you down, ask your carrier for an exemption. Many carriers have dropped some or all of their referral processes. The carriers are realizing that the vast majority of referral requests are never denied, and this process costs them staff time, too.

23. **Go electronic.** Electronic claims submissions means better use of staff and faster cash flow. Electronic payment remittance and funds transfer means less staff time spent on payment posting, more staff time spent on other duties, such as insurance follow up, and faster cash flow.

24. **Go international.** Technology has made the world a global marketplace, so consider yourself in it. Can a company in India process your transcription faster and cheaper? Explore opportunities to reduce expenses – sometimes dramatically – by looking overseas for services.

25. **Reduce your storage costs.** Scan all of the old records that you have to keep — and pay to store — medical records, explanation of benefits, charge tickets, sign-in lists, phone messages. The storage cost of several dozen CD-ROMs is exponentially cheaper than a storage facility for thousands of records.

With creativity and determination, you can find ways to cut costs in your practice.

Chapter 11

SUMMING UP

By identifying each stage of the patient encounter – from the moment a new patient calls your practice to his or her exit after the visit is concluded – you can affect change. By embracing the concept of viewing your physician's time as the practice's greatest asset and knowing the value of identifying costs and overhead, you can create an environment in which each patient encounter provides an ideal outcome for your patient in terms of customer service and your practice in terms of earnings.

Let's review the primary lessons that I hope you learned from the book:

- Your physicians' and midlevel providers' time is critical to maximizing earnings. Make them — and the systems surrounding them — more efficient to create a better bottom line.

- Real-time work processing is more efficient than batching work. Look at the processes in which you are batching work (dictation, scheduling, charge entry, etc.) and convert them to real-time work.

- Eliminating non-value-added processes can enhance customer service and lead to practice efficiency. Review processes to reduce the components that don't add value to you or your customers.

- Many medical practices have built systems that work well for their owners but, often, not for their customers. You can, and should, have systems that work for both. Explore ways to make your practice's patient flow process more patient-friendly.

- Technology is often under-utilized in the patient encounter. Seek the deployment of technology that can work for you and your patients.

- There is no "right way" to run a medical practice. Stay focused on the patient to create a patient-friendly environment in which your patients are loyal. This effort will pay for itself over and over again.

Mastering patient flow is indeed achievable, but for those practices that do reach that goal, the next challenge will be complacency. In some ways complacency is the greatest challenge of all. Once your practice believes the "ideal" has been achieved, it's time to start experimenting to make it better.

With new concepts of resource allocation and new technology on the horizon, the field of medical practice continues to be dynamic. Operating a practice will never be an easy task, but working toward the ideal patient flow process can bring a host of opportunities and rewards.

Additional Resources

Books

Ambulatory Care Management, 3rd Edition, by Austin Ross, Jr., MPH, FACMPE, Stephen J. Williams, ScD, and Ernest J. Pavlock, PhD, CPA, Delmar Publishers, available from Medical Group Management Association, 1998

Assessment Manual for Medical Groups, 4th Edition by Darrell L. Schryver, DPA (editor), Medical Group Management Association, 2002

Financial Management for Medical Groups, 2nd Edition by Ernest J. Pavlock, PhD, CPA, Medical Group Management Association Center for Research, 2000

The Goal by Eliyahu M. Goldratt, North River Press, 1985

Lean Thinking by James Womack and Daniel Jones, Simon and Schuster, 1996

Operating Policies and Procedures 2nd Edition by Bette Warn, CMPE and Elizabeth Woodcock, FACMPE, Medical Group Management Association, 2002

Perfect Practice for an Efficient Physician by Sherry Delio, MPA, Medical Group Management Association, 1999

Reinventing Medical Practice: Care Delivery that Satisfies Doctors, Patients and the Bottom Line by R. Clay Burchell, Howard L. Smith and Neill F. Piland, DrPH, Medical Group Management Association, 2002

Rightsizing: Appropriate Staffing for your Medical Practice by Deborah Walker, MBA, FACMPE and Dave Gans, MHSA, CMPE, Medical Group Management Association, 2003

Service Management: Operations, Strategy and Information Technology by James A. Fitzsimmons and Mona J. Fitzsimmons, Irwin McGraw-Hill, 1998

The Service Profit Chain by James L. Heskett, W. Earl Sasser Jr. and Leonard A. Schlesinger, The Free Press, 1997

Stop Managing Costs by James P. Mozena, Charles E. Emerick and Steven C. Black, American Society for Quality, 1999

Associations/Institutes

The Advisory Board Company, The Watergate, 600 New Hampshire, N.W., Washington, DC 20037, 202-672-5600, www.advisoryboard company.com

American College of Medical Practice Executives, 104 Inverness Terrace East, Englewood, CO, 80112, 877-275-6462,www.mgma.com/acmpe

American College of Physician Executives, 4890 West Kennedy Boulevard, Suite 200, Tampa, FL 33609, 800-562-8088, www.acpe.org

American Medical Group Association, 1422 Duke Street, Alexandria, VA 22314, 703-838-0033, www.amga.org

American Medical Association, 515 North State Street, Chicago, IL 60610, 312-464-5000, www.ama-assn.org

American Medical Informatics Association, 4915 St. Elmo Avenue, Suite 401, Bethesda, MD 20814, 301-657-1291, www.amia.org

Healthcare Financial Management Association, Two Westbrook Corporate Center, Suite 700, Westchester, IL 60154-5700, 800-252-HFMA, www.hfma.org

Institute for Healthcare Improvement, 375 Longwood Avenue, 4th Floor, Boston, MA 02215, 617-754-4800, www.ihi.org

Medical Group Management Association, 104 Inverness Terrace East, Englewood, CO, 80112, 877-ASK-MGMA, www.mgma.com

Professional Association of Health Care Office Managers, 461 East Ten Mile Road, Pensacola, FL 32534, 800-451-9311, www.pahcom.com

Specialty Societies and Associations (complete listing found at www.ama-assn.org)

State Medical Societies (complete listing found at www.ama-assn.org)

Benchmarking

MGMA *Coding Profile Sourcebook*

MGMA *Cost Survey Report*

MGMA *Management Compensation Survey Report*

MGMA *Performance and Practices of Successful Medical Groups*

Physcape Coding and Productivity Benchmarking for Medical Practices (MGMA)

MGMA *Physician Compensation and Production Survey Report*

Physician Socioeconomic Statistics (AMA)

Others

Journal of Ambulatory Care Management

Journal of Medical Practice Management

MGMA *Connexion*™

Medical Economics

The Physician's Advisory

Physicians Practice: The Business Journal for Physicians

Index